YOGA
MAMA

Also by Linda Sparrowe

The Woman's Book of Yoga and Health
(with Patricia Walden)

YOGA MAMA

The Practitioner's Guide to Prenatal Yoga

Linda Sparrowe

Photography by Sarah Keough

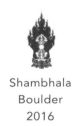

Shambhala
Boulder
2016

The information in this book is not intended as a substitute for personalized instruction and advice from an experienced yoga instructor. The reader should consult a physician before beginning this or any yoga practice or exercise program. Shambhala Publications and the author are not responsible for any adverse effects or consequences resulting directly or indirectly from the use of any of the suggestions discussed in this book.

    If you experience pain or injuries during or after these practices, it may indicate a problem that requires the attention of your physician.

Shambhala Publications, Inc.
4720 Walnut St.
Boulder, Colorado 80301
www.shambhala.com

9 8 7 6 5 4 3 2

Printed in United States of America

♾ This edition is printed on acid-free paper that meets the American National Standards Institute Z39.48 Standard.
♻ Shambhala makes every effort to print on recycled paper.
For more information please visit www.shambhala.com.

Shambhala Publications is distributed worldwide by Penguin Random House, Inc., and its subsidiaries.

Designed by Allison Meierding

Library of Congress Cataloging-in-Publication Data

Sparrowe, Linda.
Yoga mama: the practitioner's guide to prenatal yoga / Linda Sparrowe.
pages cm
ISBN 978-1-61180-130-9 (paperback)
1. Exercise for pregnant women. 2. Hatha yoga. 3. Prenatal care. 4. Postnatal care.
I. Title.
RG558.7.S63 2015
618.2′44—dc23
2014042264

CONTENTS

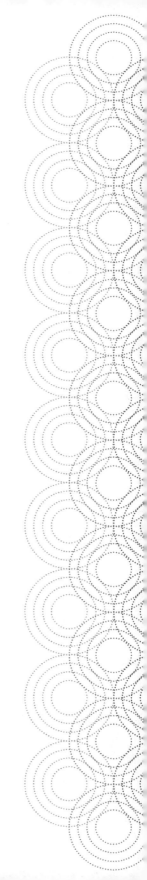

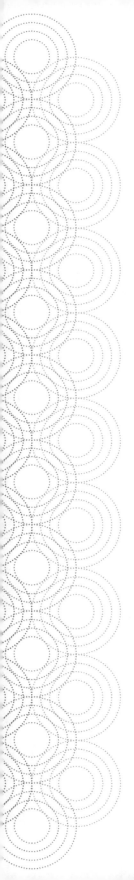

A DEEP BOW: ACKNOWLEDGMENTS

In putting together my team of *Yoga Mama* contributors, I chose women steeped in the yoga tradition and the inner workings of the body-mind who passionately believe that yoga can give us the tools we need to give birth joyfully and mindfully; their commitment elevates this offering. Elena Brower, Stephanie Snyder, Jane Austin, Melissa Williams, Margi Young, De West, Dustienne Miller, and Kate Hanley: I bow to your wisdom, patience, generosity, and your thoughtful sequencing. Jane Austin, thank you for taking time to read so much of the manuscript and offer such thoughtful suggestions. I shall miss our long phone conversations—who else could flit from the Yoga Sutra to "down there" so seamlessly? Dustienne, many thanks to you and your colleague Jessica McKinny for patiently explaining the workings of the pelvic floor. Niika Quistgard, Dr. Claudia Welch, and Kathryn Templeton, learning from you how invaluable ayurveda is for a healthy pregnancy and a joyous birth gave such depth to this book! To the many friends and yogis who recounted their birthing stories, thank you for your generosity to all women on the yoga mama path. And to Dr. Sarah Buckley, I'm indebted to you for sharing your knowledge of the inner workings of the body, gleaned not just from your medical research but also from your own at-home birthing experiences.

This book would never have come into being without the vision and enthusiasm of Sara Bercholz at Shambhala Publications and Mary Taylor of the Yoga Workshop. Thank you both for believing in me and encouraging me to find my voice and share my own wisdom without apology. And kudos to my editors, Rochelle Bourgault, who exhibited the perfect blend of gentleness and exactitude, and Beth Frankl, who graciously took this book to the finish line.

Sarah Forbes Keough, I love the photographs! Thank you for such a joyful collaboration and for helping everything stay in focus—both figuratively and literally. And Jenn Falk, Emily Reardon, Emily Weibel, Sara Bercholz, and Rochelle Bourgault—thank you for gracing the pages with your radiant selves and beautiful postures.

This book benefited greatly from my younger daughter, Megan's, own pregnancy. Thanks, Megan—good timing! Being part of that nine-month journey (and beyond), doing yoga together, breathing together, sharing thoughts and feelings, and holding your darling baby boy in my arms are gifts I will cherish forever.

Finally, I could never have written this book without my practice, the wisdom of the ancient seers, and the generosity of my own teachers. May yoga continue to guide you all inward and teach you to trust your innate ability to give birth to your baby and to yourself.

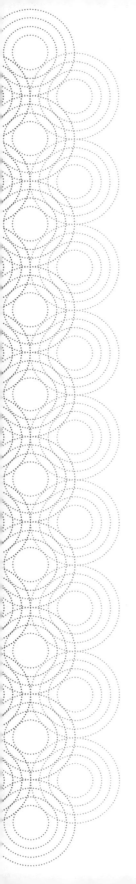

INTRODUCTION

When I first started writing about yoga and pregnancy years ago, I focused on how to listen deeply and stay open to the experience of sharing your body with another being. That translated to a lot of sitting around, meditating, and chanting with eyes closed, or lying around in luscious restorative poses supported with straps, bolsters, and eye pillows. All of those things do, indeed, yield a sense of connection and a means of self-reflection that no amount of busyness or working out could replicate. But women wanted more. They didn't want to give up their practice, sidelining Sun Salutations and backbends in favor of nine months of Savasana. They wanted the yoga they did every day to continue to be an integral part of their lives.

So I decided to write this book to help women do just that. I dug deep into both of my prenatal experiences and found that I had actually been happiest when I took the time to move, stretch, balance, and ground, as well as rest. I love to dance—it makes me feel engaged with my body in a completely joyful way—so I kept dancing. Yoga makes me feel strong and centered, so I kept practicing. Many of my students and other women I spoke to felt the same way. For them, moving through their vinyasa practice kept their morning sickness at bay and gave them a sense of normalcy. So a book with flowing sequences seemed to fit the bill.

But then I remembered more. My two pregnancies were also liberally sprinkled with days of mind-numbing fatigue; bouts of queasiness, back pain, and indigestion; and waves of anxiety and doubt. Some days, the idea of stepping onto my mat at all made me want to hurl. When I told other women about this, they nodded knowingly and shared their own stories. One well-known teacher even admitted that she didn't want to do any asanas through most of her pregnancy and that made her feel like she had somehow failed as a yogi.

Obviously, a book made up solely of strong vinyasa sequences wouldn't work. The last thing I wanted was for women to judge their own experiences harshly or jump into something they felt was inappropriate. But the question that most yoga practitioners ask almost as soon as they learn they're pregnant is still an important one: *Do I have to give up my practice?* My answer: *It depends*. It depends on what your body (and your baby) needs at any given moment. You'll no doubt give it up, take it back, and give it up again multiple times during your pregnancy and your postpartum adventures.

My advice is if your usual practice feels good, do it. But don't hold on to it if it doesn't. A strong yoga practice, with plenty of backbending and inverting, throughout your pregnancy may feel great. It can help you build physical strength, confidence in yourself, and an emotional bond with your baby, and it even helps alleviate anxiety and fatigue. However, if you can barely get out of bed for the first few months, a flowing practice is the last thing your body needs. Gentle breathing techniques, along with shedding plenty of tears and eating saltines, may become your new practice. I want women to know that both responses—and everything in between—are appropriate. Both are *yoga*. All is yoga. They cease being yoga, of course, when the mind's insistence on what *should* be trumps the body's need for what *must* be.

I wrote this book to offer as many choices as possible. *Yoga Mama* is divided into chapters that include all three trimesters, pelvic floor advice, and the "fourth trimester"—the first three months of your postbirthing life with baby. Within each chapter you'll find the following:

* Sequences from a stellar group of pre- and postnatal yoga teachers, with plenty of advice and suggestions on how to modify your practice
* Breathing techniques for everything from morning sickness and fatigue to labor and birthing
* Short meditation sequences, designed to help you listen more intently to your baby's needs and your body's subtle and not-so-subtle cues
* A feature I call "the inside scoop"—a guide to what's happening in your body and with your baby at all stages of pregnancy

• Information and advice from midwives, integrative doctors, and ayurvedic specialists on what to eat, how to prepare your mind and body for a natural birth, and when to reach out for help

• Teachings from the ancient texts of yoga and ayurveda that may help support you during your journey (Although many of these teachings apply all through the pregnancy, birthing, and post-partum stages, I've chosen to place each one where I think it will resonate the most.)

An all-star group of guest teachers offers sequences for the book:

• **Melissa Williams**, the owner of the Yoga Junction studio in Louisville, Colorado, shares the mini sequences she's designed for fatigue, hip and pelvic pain, and indigestion.

• **Elena Brower**, an internationally known yoga teacher, takes you through a now-that-you're-pregnant series, grounded in plenty of self-inquiry and designed to open up space to welcome your baby.

• **Stephanie Snyder**, one of the Bay Area's most popular teachers, offers a fairly energetic second-trimester sequence, peppered with suggested modifications for those days when you feel the need to take things down a notch.

• **Margi Young**, an OM yoga teacher originally from New York City, keeps the momentum going throughout the third trimester, while acknowledging that your belly and your flagging energy may impede your ability to flow from one pose to the other.

• **Jane Austin**—childbirth educator, prenatal teacher, and creator of MamaTree prenatal teacher training in San Francisco—focuses attention on the pelvic floor, a critical part of the labor and birthing puzzle that can mean the difference between a long, difficult experience and a joyous one.

• **De West**, a Boulder, Colorado–based prenatal teacher, moves you through the labor and birthing process with partner poses and breath-centric techniques.

• **Dustienne Miller**, a Boston yoga teacher and physical therapist, offers advice and poses to help you knit everything back together after your baby arrives and return to your mat safely.

• **Kate Hanley**, a yoga author and life coach, chimes in with much-needed advice for the fourth trimester, including how to tailor your yoga practice to help you sleep, calm your nerves, and even encourage your milk to flow.

• **Sarah Buckley**, MD, an integrative health expert, finds room within the medical field for mindful yoga and conscious breathing.

Keep Your Move On

In every trimester, I recommend doing some kind of physical practice, even when you're not feeling up to a full-fledged sequence. That's because physical practice helps us know and trust the body's capabilities at any given moment and activates what yogis call compassionate self-observation. Just rooting around in your muscles, joints, and tissues—as well as your mind and heart—helps you notice any physical or emotional resistance, tightness, or blockages that prevent the prana, or life force, from flowing freely.

What you do can change from day to day. You may feel like doing something as simple as walking around the block or slow dancing around the room, or you may be up for committing to something as full as a ninety-minute class. A very modified, slow-flow Sun Salutation, or a combination of vinyasa and restorative poses may also fit the bill. Whatever practice you choose, pay close attention to your breath, sending the exhalation to an area that needs to release a bit more or feel a tender touch.

Yoga is indeed a physical practice, a body-based meditation, but it's also so much more. Yoga brings the mind into the experience and helps us to "live all the details of our lives," as Pema Chödrön once said about Buddhist practice. This makes it an invaluable ally in pregnancy. Every pregnancy is different; every birth happens exactly the way it's supposed to, which makes every prenatal yoga practice unique. Yoga asks women to trust in the process and to stay on their own mats, as it were, rooted in their own experience. Through your physical practice and conscious breath work, you can create a bond with your baby that will help you birth her into being.

I wrote this book to encourage women to stay true to their practice—to give them permission, in a way, to continue moving through their before-pregnancy sequences. But to be truthful, I had a more important message in mind. I want this book to be a call to mindful action. I want yoga practice to facilitate the most natural, most mindful childbirth experience possible. I also want yoga to help every woman trust her own instincts and awaken her *vijnanamaya kosha*, her intuitive wisdom, so that she can override the negative, fear-based, and often unsolicited advice she gets that grips her imagination and can cause her to make choices that may not be the kindest or healthiest ones.

Mindful action asks us to embrace our practice wholeheartedly as being much more than exercise with yoga shapes. It's more than rocking three sweaty Surya Namaskar As and three Bs first thing in the morning. In the vinyasa classes I teach, I remind my students that under all the confusion, fear, or impatience they may feel on any given day lies an inner knowing untouched by judgments or uncertainty. When we have the opportunity to spend time in our body, gently and tenderly getting to know ourselves, we learn what it needs to be healthy, happy, and whole. We learn not to impose our thinking mind's advice on the actions of the body.

You've probably experienced this in yoga class. Do you ever notice, for instance, that you can balance so much better when you stop thinking about *how* to balance, where to place your foot, or why you never seem to stay up as long as the person next to you? When my mind tries to control my physical practice instead of taking cues from my body, I get in trouble. I fall over or, worse, hurt myself.

This same principle applies to giving birth, the primal forces of which happen in the deepest recesses of our brain, blessedly removed from linear thinking and emotional reactions. By learning to get out of your own way and surrender to your deepest instincts, you can trust your capacity to give birth gracefully, naturally, and even joyfully. Yoga allows us to meet our hopes as well as our fears, our joys as well as our sorrows, like old friends, knowing they all live within us but accepting that none of them defines us. We learn to bring our whole self to every moment on the wave of the breath.

But you can't do all this alone. Yoga is the inner coach of your team of birthing experts. From that place of inner reflection and practical knowledge that yoga provides, you must create a team of people who share your commitment to birthing naturally and joyfully. A midwife, a doula, and a loving partner or trusted friend can help "see us into being," to borrow a Stephen Cope phrase. There are aspects of ourselves we cannot see or feel, he told me, "without the mirroring of another, trusted being" who allows us to see ourselves in their reflection. This "active and co-creative seeing" is exactly what we need to trust our ability to surrender into the mystery of childbirth.

Even though you can't make your pregnancy and birthing experience happen exactly the way you want it to, surrounding yourself with "trusted beings" will help create the conditions that will give you and your baby the best chance of having the experience you envision. The sad truth is the medicalization of pregnancy and childbirth can sometimes overwhelm women with the best intentions and cause them to make choices—accepting pain medication, inducing labor, having a cesarean birth—they may not need or want to make. The good news, of course, is when you have a midwife or doula advocate for you in a hospital setting, the incidence of intervention (such as pain meds, induced labor, and cesarean births) decreases dramatically.

My loving advice to you: Keep practicing and surround yourself with people who believe in you and whom you trust completely. Yoga will give you the physical strength to endure potentially hours of labor and intense sensations and the self-awareness that you have everything you need to give birth. Most important, it teaches you to let go of the thinking mind and surrender to the primordial wisdom you share with your foremothers, diving deep into the mammalian brain's hormonal birthing brew. Your loving team of experts will stand beside you, fielding questions and removing all obstacles, so you can partner with your baby to create a smooth passage from your belly into your arms.

YOGA MAMA

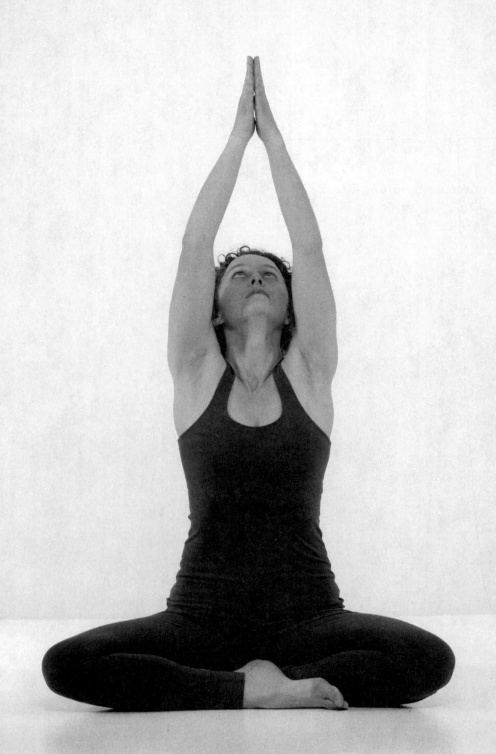

1.

FIRST TRIMESTER

Welcoming and Accepting
From Conception to Thirteen Weeks

Sequences by Elena Brower
and Melissa Williams

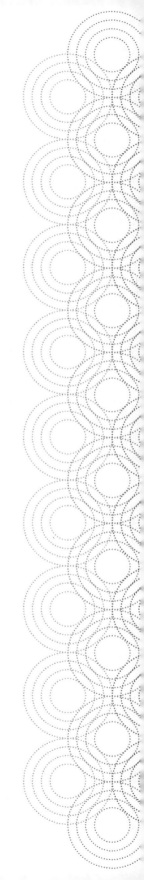

The first time I got pregnant, I had no idea what was wrong with me. I thought I was suffering from some sort of prolonged PMS or sheer exhaustion from starting a new job. My husband suggested I take one of those home pregnancy tests, just in case. It was positive. Suddenly everything made sense—my sore breasts, my fatigue, and even my slightly off-kilter sense of balance. Three years later, pregnant again, I felt the physical and emotional changes immediately. What a difference three more years of a yoga and meditation practice made. I felt much more aligned with my body and sensitive to any fluctuations in my physical, mental, and emotional states.

Both times, I felt the need to keep the news between my husband and me. Initially I resisted seeking advice, buying books on the subject, or even making a doctor's appointment. I simply wanted to feel what it was like to be pregnant without anyone else's spin on it, without the benefit of other people's experiences. My experience and decisions are hardly unique. Anyone who has spent time on a yoga mat getting to know her body understands that there's a certain beauty in listening internally, experiencing her body from the inside before reaching outward.

I read once in a yoga book for beginners that everyone should come to yoga open, empty, and bare; that is, with an open mind, empty belly, and bare feet. Playing off that advice a little bit, I can see how pregnancy—and ultimately labor, birthing, and even parenting—can become more meaningful if we stay open, empty, and bare. An open mind helps you listen to what your body needs and what it has to teach you instead of enforcing your will (or someone else's) on it. It lets you be open to whatever arises, paying attention without trying to control, compartmentalize, judge, or change anything.

Emptying your mind of any preconceived notions of what should or shouldn't happen when you're pregnant will help you notice what actually is happening. Suzuki Roshi, revered Zen master and author of *Zen Mind, Beginner's Mind*, says, "If your mind is empty, it is always ready for anything; it is open to everything." Being bare means being willing to stand naked in the face of the mystery, stripped of judgments. In other words, yoga can help you stay open to the full experience of this pregnancy without filtering it through what you think you already know.

The Inside Scoop

So what should you be paying attention to at this point? Knowing what's going on inside your body, beginning with the first trimester, can help you figure that out. Then you can create the type of practice that makes the most sense physically and emotionally. You'll also begin to understand and accept the sometimes odd "side effects" that may present themselves during the first trimester: tender breasts, frequent trips to the bathroom, gastric distress, nausea, mind-numbing fatigue, and that weird stitch in your side—which, by the way, is your uterus expanding and moving into place.

The moment your partner's sperm breaks through to your egg, your body begins to prepare room in the womb for the fertilized egg to take up residence and receive ample nourishment so it can grow. The tiny embryonic cell will take about three weeks to make its journey down the fallopian tubes and into the uterus, all the while multiplying and dividing. When it gets to the uterus, it will adhere to the uterine wall as a collection of cells called a blastocyst. Some of these cells develop into the fetus; others go on to form the placenta.

The blastocyst's occupancy is tenuous at best, so all systems—from the brain and the heart to the lungs and the adrenal glands that sit atop the kidneys—shift their collective focus to ensure a successful implantation. Your immune system slows down to prevent your body from rejecting the blastocyst as a foreign intruder; your musculoskeletal system allows the muscle tissue to relax and the joints to loosen so the uterus can move into position and stretch and grow along with the baby. Your endocrine system produces a hormone called human chorionic gonadotropin (hCG) that keeps the ovaries churning out progesterone until the placenta can take over. This prevents the body from shedding its uterine lining—and its occupant—prematurely. Blood pressure drops so the heart can pump additional fluid; along with a huge influx of hormones, this thickens and stabilizes the uterine lining. The hormone progesterone relaxes the smooth muscle—the muscle in the uterus (as well as in the gastrointestinal tract and blood vessels) that involuntarily contracts to push things out of the body—thereby preventing premature labor. Of course, all this excess progesterone also causes gastrointestinal distress and sore breasts, which are often your first clue that you're pregnant.

Once it's fully formed (at about three months), the placenta produces enough progesterone to support and nourish the fetus, keep the uterine lining intact, and prevent the uterus from contracting. It also uses enormous amounts of estrogen from your—and your baby's—adrenal glands. The estrogen and progesterone combine to keep your smooth muscle tissue relaxed, so your uterus can expand and your body can accommodate the increased demand for excess fluids and blood.

Taking an Internal Inventory

If you've had a long-time yoga practice, you may sense the subtle (and not-so-subtle) changes in your body even before the little circle shows up on a urine-based pregnancy test and the fertilized egg has made its descent. As soon as you feel those changes, you should begin to shift your awareness even more deeply inward. Why? Because, as the ancient ayurvedic texts say, "The earlier the event, the deeper the impression." Western doctors tend to agree, and several studies show that drinking alcohol, doing drugs, and even being in a stressful relationship—especially in the earliest stages of pregnancy—can have a deleterious effect on the tiny being in utero. But according to ayurveda, the reverse is also true: everything healthy and mindful a woman does leaves an equally deep and lasting impression.

Of course, if you weren't aware of your pregnancy until weeks or more after it began, don't worry. You still have plenty of time to influence your baby's life in a positive way. You just need to live as consciously and compassionately as you can. Luckily, according to yoga (and Buddhist) philosophy, that is a mother's true nature.

My friend Claudia Welch, who is an ayurvedic practitioner and author, has a spiritual teacher who used to tell his students to do their meditation practice lovingly and not think of it as a burden. For Claudia, the obvious meaning behind her guru's words was that love and longing pull us closer to the Divine, while indifference renders our *sadhana* (spiritual practices) little more than exercises in discipline. The same thing can be said about the way we approach our yoga practice and our pregnancy. If you come to the mat with the intention of creating a deeper, more loving connection with your body, you'll have an easier time noticing what's happening and even participating in this amazing time of transition. Indeed, if you commit to this journey as early and as mindfully as possible, giving it your heartfelt attention, you'll not only nourish the divine life growing inside you, but you will also be pulled closer to (and able to trust in) your own innate goodness as a mother.

Adjusting Your Yoga Practice

What does all of this internal activity mean for your yoga practice? Should you stop completely and wait for everything to settle into place or consign yourself to the restorative world of blankets, blocks, and bolsters for the next twelve weeks? Neither, unless you want to. Continue doing what you've been doing (with a few modifications), as long as it feels good. However, if you have a history of miscarriage or begin spotting, ask your midwife or doctor for advice before you resume your practice. She may recommend you wait until the second trimester. Of course, if you are incapacitated by nausea, fatigue, or other physical discomfort, yoga may be the furthest thing from your mind right now, and that's fine, too.

Continuing your yoga practice doesn't necessarily mean jumping back on your yoga mat or doing your sequences as though nothing has changed. Even if you have tons of energy and your usual practice still feels great, everything *has* changed: everything you do from now on, you'll do in concert with your baby. Sometimes that means slowing down your practice, staying with the breath, and directing your attention to your body in new ways; other times it means doing a strong vinyasa practice; and still other times it means breaking out the blankets, blocks, and bolsters.

Staying Strong

As a committed Ashtanga practitioner, Jeanie Manchester saw no reason to stop doing her regular practice when she got pregnant. She didn't suffer from morning sickness, and doing yoga actually helped her fatigue levels. But the way she moved through her sequence was different. She was much more aware of the subtle changes in her body. "I was cautious whenever I felt a pull or a weird stretch," Jeanie says, "because I knew my body was making room for my baby, and I needed and wanted to listen." She included everything from Sun Salutations to Headstand and from Handstand at the wall to full backbends the first three months. Physically, Jeanie felt strong. "All the [primary series] standing poses made me feel like if I could hold them, I could endure anything—even labor and birthing," she says. No one would recommend introducing strong inversions and backbends in the first trimester if you don't already do them as part of your regular practice, but there's no reason to give them up now if they feel good, unless you have a history of miscarriage.

Slowing Down

Sometimes shifting your practice to a slower pace can help you stay in touch with your emotions or sort through some complex feelings. Elena Brower, co-author of *Art of Attention* and creator of Teach.Yoga, an online resource by teachers for teachers, found this to be the case. Early in her pregnancy, she experienced not only profound joy but palpable fear: Was she truly capable of being responsible for someone else's life? Could she really mother such an innocent being? By practicing yoga, meditating, and doing Reiki, she was able to face those fears without judgment and simply let them go. "My practice helped me understand and embrace the power of the bond my baby and I were already forging and prepared me for the journey ahead," she says.

Some women (especially first-time mamas) choose not to do much physical yoga during the first trimester, focusing on their meditation or pranayama practice instead. Sometimes those first few months feel too precarious, and women want to wait to make sure the little fertilized egg has firmly implanted itself for the long haul. Others—let's get real—feel far too sick to even think about bopping up and down in a vinyasa class. Claudia Cummins, a long-time yoga teacher from Ohio, says she just couldn't bring herself to do yoga in the beginning; morning sickness left her feeling weak and queasy almost all the time. "My yoga morphed into a slow walk down the street and back," she says. Even after she felt better, she found herself yearning to be still, as she describes rather poetically, "My yoga practice was slow, round, and very close to the ground."

As a general rule, you need to modify or shelve only those poses that no longer feel good. Of course, that list of poses may change depending on how your body responds from one day (or even one moment) to the next. Whether you continue your regularly scheduled practice like Jeanie or focus mostly on pranayama to keep from hurling like Claudia, or craft a practice somewhere in between like Elena, the most important modification you can make is to place your attention less on the physical and more on the breath, which will keep you anchored and tuned inward. By creating conditions that are conducive to self-discovery, you will get to know yourself on a much more intimate level, and you'll learn to figure out what makes sense for you and what feels right. This place of inner knowing or intuitive wisdom can do more than help you gain the most benefit from your yoga practice. It can also guide you in knowing and caring for your child and yourself during and after your pregnancy. Accessing your intuition allows you to sift through all the information coming at you from doctors, books, nurses, midwives, and well-meaning friends; absorb it all; and find what works for you. Yoga can give you a sense of clarity, confidence, and compassion, all of which you need to become the best mother you can possibly be. And you can get all that whether you are continuing your usual asana practice or lying over a bolster in the dark with an eye pillow to block out queasy distractions. How? By always coming back to the breath, paying attention to the quality of your inhalations and exhalations, and perhaps turning to the deeper teachings of this ancient practice.

Returning to the Roots of Practice

Patanjali's Yoga Sutra, compiled as long ago as 200 B.C.E., is one of the most important—and certainly the most well-known—philosophical texts in yoga. It offers advice and practices that you may find useful all through your pregnancy, but especially during the first few months when you may be sorting through conflicting information and complex emotions. Most yoga practitioners are aware of the *yamas* and *niyamas* (precepts for how we interact in the world and how we care for ourselves) and how they guide us toward becoming more self-aware, more awake to what's happening around us, and more attuned to our own true nature. Patanjali also presents three concepts that helped me find my own path through the birthing journey: *tapas* (action or discipline), *svadhyaya* (self-reflection), and *ishvara pranidhana* (surrender). Exploring these on the mat during the first few months may help you clarify their meaning and take them off the mat and into your everyday experiences.

TAPAS: AN INTENSE COMMITMENT

From the moment you announce your pregnancy, you may find yourself inundated with more advice and information than you can possibly process. How do you sort through it all? How can you even know what's good advice and what's not? Start by practicing tapas. *Tapas* means a whole slew of things: discipline, intense focus, heat, even simplicity or austerity. When we commit to practicing anything with fierce determination, when we choose to show up whether we feel like it or not, when we face our fears head-on, or when we muster enough willpower to stay the course no matter what's ahead—that's tapas.

You already experience tapas, often associated with internal heat, whenever you do a vigorous vinyasa practice. This heat allows you to release tension from or tightness in your body during practice. When I was about three months pregnant, I went to an all-day yoga intensive led by a well-known yoga teacher, who had us all stand in Tadasana (Mountain Pose) for thirty minutes. At first, of course, it was no big deal. I focused on my posture and executing the finer points of the pose. But after about fifteen minutes, I thought, *There's no way I can do this. My whole body hurts. I feel dizzy. I'm bored. I want to do something else now*. As the intensity of the experience mounted, I began to notice a lot of tension in my shoulders and neck and cramping in my legs and feet. So I decided I would try one more thing before I bailed: I would release all effort that wasn't necessary to stand there and see if that helped. And it did. By engaging my muscles just enough to keep me upright, the pose felt manageable—not fabulous or even comfortable, but manageable. Those thirty minutes on the mat gave me a glimpse of how I could use tapas later on during labor and birth. I was really happy I had that experience so early in my pregnancy. I didn't have to worry so much, wondering if I had the willpower to hold steady when things got difficult, and equally important, I discovered that I could use my body's internal heat to melt away physical and mental tension.

Tapas can also help you show up for and negotiate any uncertainty you feel. The intense focus it brings purifies the mind because it cuts through doubt and gives you confidence to make the right decisions for you and your baby. Finally, tapas (in the sense of austerity) becomes a practice of simplicity: clearing out the clutter and shedding extraneous thoughts, actions, and information so you can dig down to a fundamental truth: you already know how to give birth. Women's bodies are hardwired to do that, and your body is no different. My friend Janice Gates, who is a yoga therapist and prenatal teacher in Marin County, California, says she embraced tapas as a way of doing "a little internal housecleaning." She found pregnancy to be the perfect time for burning up all the old stuff—judgments, fears, feelings of inadequacy, destructive habits she'd been meaning to get rid of for years—and paring down to the essentials in preparation for her new life.

SVADHYAYA: TURNING THE LENS INWARD

Of course, if you focus solely on tapas without any svadhyaya (self-awareness), you run the risk of burning yourself up along with all that extraneous stuff. Becoming so completely fixated on orchestrating the perfect pose or even the perfect birthing experience may lead to self-aggression, injury, and oftentimes disappointment and heartache.

Every pregnancy is different, and any action you take as a pregnant mama must be right for your particular needs and circumstances, as well as your baby's. So the next step, as the Yoga Sutra teaches us, is to inquire into the nature of the self: svadhyaya. One aspect of such self-inquiry, studying the texts, can take on a dual meaning during this time. Taking refuge in the Yoga Sutra, the Bhagavad Gita, or any other texts (ancient or contemporary) that resonate with you or seeking advice from a spiritual teacher may offer you insight and comfort. Conferring with or reading the advice of prenatal experts can also serve you well. Do you have prenatal books you gravitate toward or inspirational texts that inspire you? Read them. Are there particular experts whose knowledge you value or wisdom you seek? Study with them. But be discerning or you'll find yourself more stressed and confused than ever.

Some women find comfort in reading everything they can get their hands on about pregnancy and birthing. Others seek the advice of friends who have already had babies. My daughter had planned to have a natural birth, so during her pregnancy she focused on gathering information that would prepare her for that experience. She knew exactly what she wanted to do and didn't want to be deterred by advice that would pull her off task. Pam England, the author of *Birthing Within*, calls this "modern knowledge," a way of hunting and gathering that can help us navigate the complexities of modern-day, medicalized birthing options; natural at-home births; and everything in between.

Svadhyaya also means to reflect on what you've read and heard. There's a lot of information out there. Some good and some not so good. You'll need to commit to paying attention to what feels true for you and put the rest aside—just like you do in your daily yoga practice. Above all, don't begin your journey by getting so wrapped up in the research that you forget to experience the joy of discovery. Begin by trusting your own instincts. Relish the process. You know better than anyone else what feels good and what doesn't, what you need in order to nourish and nurture yourself and your little one. If you commit to self-awareness now, it'll be easier to draw from it later on in your pregnancy. Remember, when things get too overwhelming, take a breather and repeat this mantra: *I have everything I need to birth this beautiful baby. I am a capable and loving mother.*

And then practice yoga—whatever that looks like right now. No doubt your practice will change repeatedly throughout your pregnancy, as well it should. Right now, pay close attention to your breath and the quality of your experience as you move through the different poses, and ask yourself questions like, *What does my body need right now? Is the class too fast for me today or not quite enough? Is the pain I feel in my knee harmful? Does this sequence make room for my baby? Should I take a nap or take a walk instead?* In other words, doing yoga throughout your pregnancy, even in the earliest weeks, will give you the opportunity to reflect on your experience as it is happening and to shift it as necessary.

Can I go more deeply into this pose, or do I need to back off? What is my baby feeling as I hold this posture? This is svadhyaya, or primordial knowing, in action. Discipline (tapas) softened with compassion brings nonjudgmental self-awareness (svadhyaya).

ISHVARA PRANIDHANA: TRUST AND SURRENDER

Prenatal expert Jane Austin puts it this way: "Yoga keeps us honest. When we acknowledge how and what we are feeling, we honor our experience. From this place of honoring, we can let go of expectations or judgment." That is the practice of surrender, or what the Yoga Sutra calls *ishvara pranidhana*. Svadhyaya helps ground us in our own experience so we're not influenced by everyone else's hopes and, even worse, fears. Practicing ishvara pranidhana invites us to let go of anything that doesn't ring true and simply sit with what is. Pregnancy can be a powerful time to look within and find or cultivate trust. By trusting

Elena's Story

Looking back on my first few months of pregnancy, I felt like I had to hack my life daily, to break some secret code and completely change something about how I was thinking or feeling, and to face the real fear about my ability to be responsible for someone else's life. I had a few weeks of being really, really sick, and it was downright humbling. I needed to connect to my body as often as possible, and there were a few ways I was able to do that: yoga, Reiki, and meditation.

Pregnancy showed me my connection to the planet, to the magic of evolution, and to my sacred role in the process. When I speak about pregnancy, it is with such care and gratitude. Pregnancy continues to inform my practice, even today. It reminds me to make daily connections to the earth, to center myself on the ground, and to feel my feet literally and figuratively. Throughout the experience, I kept finding myself in a remarkable state of reverence for all of it, even when I was depleted and super sick. Perhaps seeking and receiving that reverence is the essence of the practice during this time.

our body's ability to give birth, we can let go of the need to control the outcome with our logical brain and simply surrender to the mystery of the whole process.

Practicing yoga gives us the discipline (tapas) to stand up for ourselves and our baby, to act decisively and compassionately, to show up even when we're anxious or too sick to get out of bed, and to ask the hard questions we need answers to. It gives us the self-awareness (svadhyaya) to filter out all the noise, embrace what works for us moment to moment, and let go of what doesn't (ishvara pranidhana). Sometimes that letting go can even include relationships that don't feel good anymore or may be a little toxic.

But surrender goes beyond shedding unwelcome advice or fleeing noxious situations; it also means letting go of our attachment to any particular outcome. In this place of not knowing, we must surrender to our intuitive nature—what the Buddhists call prajna, or "best knowing." You can't make your pregnancy and birthing experience happen a certain way, but you can create conditions that give you and your baby the best chance of having the experience you envision. And find the patience to allow things to unfold as they will.

First Trimester Challenges

Some women sail through the first three months with few complaints; others can barely get out of bed. Most of us have experiences that fall somewhere in between. Regardless of where you are on the first trimester continuum, your emotions may be all over the map, bouncing back and forth between excitement and terror, confidence and confusion, especially if you've never been pregnant before. The most common physical complaints—nausea, fatigue, breast tenderness, constipation, and cramping—sound like a litany of PMS symptoms, and no wonder. Just like PMS, they appear to be the result of surging hormones. Yoga can offer ways of at least softening the intensity of these challenges, but you'll quite likely have to rearrange your idea of what doing yoga means until you feel better.

A Note of Caution

• As soon as you discover you're pregnant, stop doing twists that press against your belly. According to B.K.S. Iyengar, twists give your body the signal to squeeze and expel, and that's not the action you want during pregnancy. Open twists like Bharadvajasana (Simple Seated Twist Pose) work nicely to open your shoulders and release any tension in your back.

• If you have a history of miscarriage, shelve your yoga practice until you get through the first trimester or you get the OK from your doctor.

• Don't do poses that don't feel good—physically and intuitively.

• Don't practice in a room that's hotter than your body temperature (about 98.6°F).

• If you have an established practice, don't introduce new poses during pregnancy; stick with what you know.

• Approach all familiar poses without any preconceptions about how deeply you should go into them or how they should feel. You may find that some of your usual poses need to be modified or eliminated and some you've avoided can be reintroduced, depending on how you feel.

MORNING SICKNESS

No one knows what causes morning sickness, or why some women get it and others don't. The medical term, *nausea and vomiting in pregnancy* (NVP), pretty much says it all. You may have a wretched time in the morning, and then your symptoms ease up the rest of the day. Or your nausea may come in waves, triggered by certain smells, the motion of a car, or certain foods. Or maybe there's nothing "morning" about your sickness—it hangs on all day. That's what happened to Claudia Cummins and Stephanie Snyder. Both women had strong yoga practices before becoming pregnant and expected to maintain these practices right up until the day their babies appeared.

"Someone once showed me a photo of herself upside-down in Headstand that had been taken the day before her child was born," Claudia says. "And I thought, 'Yup, that will be me.'" Unfortunately, her baby had other plans. "I could barely eat a piece of toast, let alone stand in Triangle Pose," she says. "Mostly I wanted to lie still, and if that didn't work, I wanted to be outside." Stephanie had it even worse: she was nearly bedridden with morning sickness during her two pregnancies. For both women, yoga became simple breathing techniques to calm the stomach (and nervous system) and slow walks outside on their "good" days.

If you have less severe prenatal sickness, you can do a few standing poses and see how they feel. Tadasana (Mountain Pose), Ardha Chandrasana (Half-Moon Pose) and Vrksasana (Tree Pose) are often stabilizing and can increase circulation. To combat nausea, try exhaling into your feet to ground your energy; keep your focus (*drishti*) straight ahead; and do forward extensions rather than forward bends, which means keeping your head up instead of dropping it down.

Many theories exist to explain prenatal nausea, but no one really knows the answer. Most experts at least partially blame human chorionic gonadotropin, the hormone we discussed earlier that helps prevent the body from rejecting the fetus early on. That's a reasonable assumption, because the queasy feelings for most women begin about the same time as their hCG levels spike and then usually taper off when the hormone levels decrease. However, experts at Mayo Clinic point to the combined surge in progesterone and estrogen, which causes the stomach to empty more slowly, as the culprit for nausea. Others say the enormous amounts of estrogen a pregnant body produces may cause women to become hypersensitive to odors—so much so that certain smells can trigger the gag reflex. A sluggish digestive system and waves of anxiety could also contribute to morning sickness.

Ultimately, of course, the cause hardly matters, unless you can identify certain things that trigger an attack and avoid them. Most pregnant women simply want to know how to cope. If you literally can't keep a thing down and the nausea or vomiting becomes severe, or if you feel dizzy or faint when you stand up, give your doctor a call.

For run-of-the-mill morning sickness, you may get relief from one or more of these suggestions:

- Keep moving: even a slow, meditative walk may make you feel better.
- Practice a few standing poses (against the wall, if you feel dizzy or weak); they can sometimes help alleviate your discomfort.
- Continue any breathing practices (pranayama) that you would normally do for anxiety. Nadi Shodhana (Alternate Nostril Breathing), Ujjayi Pranayama (Victorious Breath), and Viloma Pranayama I (Interval Breathing I) may work well (see practices on page 175). For most women, five to ten minutes of Belly Breathing (with emphasis on the exhalation) is all that's required.
- If you're mobile, practice the morning sickness sequence (page 16), which includes standing poses to ground your energy, and a few resting poses.
- Keep crackers by your bed, and eat one or two before you even get up in the morning. Even though you're supposed to drink plenty of liquids, doing so first thing in the morning can some-times make you feel worse; instead, sip warm water or peppermint tea later in the day.
- Eat simple foods: apples, pears, or bananas; a little cheese on crackers (for an added bit of fat); or a handful of almonds.
- Take your prenatal vitamins just before you go to bed (instead of in the morning), because some brands can send your stomach on a roller coaster ride. You may have to try a couple of different types before you find one you can tolerate.
- Try any nonpharmaceutical that works for motion sickness: all things ginger, such as tea (crushed ginger in hot water, steeped for ten minutes), chews, biscuits, or crackers; an acupressure band around your wrist; a soothing aromatherapy stick (peppermint, lemon, or lavender are favorites); or a couple of drops of pure essential oils on a handkerchief that you carry with you.
- Alternative therapies, such as acupuncture or hypnotherapy, definitely help some women.

MY MORNING SICKNESS SEQUENCE

Do as many (or as few) of these poses as you like, moving in concert with your breath. Skip over any asanas that don't work for you, and keep your eyes open if you feel nauseous or dizzy.

Sukhasana (Easy Seated Pose) with Arm Movements

Sit in a comfortable cross-legged position. Slowly inhale as you raise your arms out to the sides and up overhead until your palms touch. Exhale as you round your back and bring your hands down to your chest, keeping your palms together. Clasp your fingers together and inhale your arms out in front of you and overhead. Exhale through your mouth as you release your arms down by your sides until your hands rest on the floor. Do this sequence 3 to 5 times.

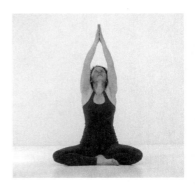
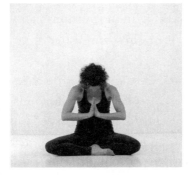
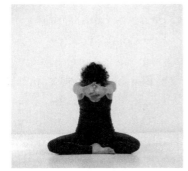
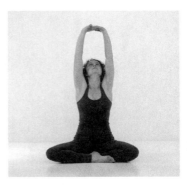
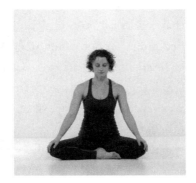

Vajrasana Surya Namaskar (Thunderbolt Sun Salutation)

Use your inhalation to initiate each movement and your exhalation to complete each movement—as slowly and mindfully as possible. Begin by sitting on your heels in Vajrasana (Thunderbolt Pose) with your hands in prayer position at your heart. Inhale as you come up to your knees and raise your arms up overhead, touching palms together. On your next exhalation, move into Balasana (Child's Pose) with your arms back by your sides. Inhale up to your hands and knees, gently arch your back and look up toward the ceiling and, as you exhale, round your back like a cat, pressing your hands into the mat. On your next inhale, rise up onto your knees once again, lifting your arms overhead and touching palms together in a gentle backbend, and exhale back down to sit on your heels. Repeat this mini vinyasa 3 to 5 times.

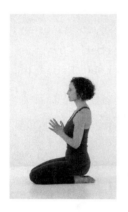 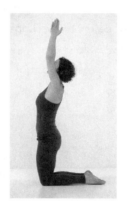 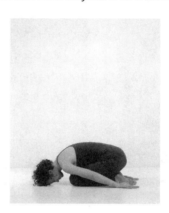 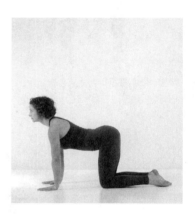

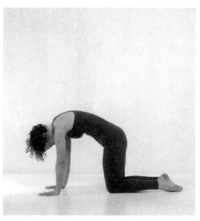 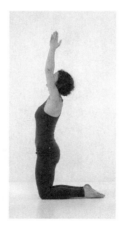 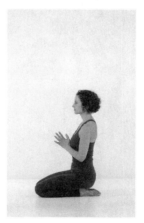

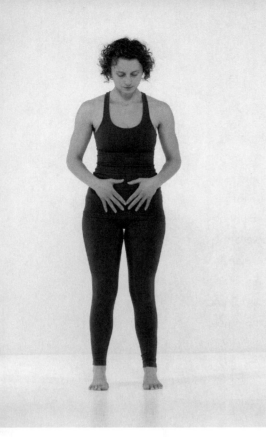

Tadasana (Mountain Pose)

Stand in Tadasana with your feet about hip-width apart. Take a moment to feel your feet on the ground and experience your relationship with gravity. Place your hands on your belly, breathing slowly and gently, keeping your eyes open and focused a few feet in front of you. If you're tired or feel nauseous, practice this pose with your back against the wall. Hold the pose for 5 full breaths, or as long as it feels soothing.

Ardha Surya Namaskar (Mini Sun Salutation)

Start in Tadasana (Mountain Pose) with your hands in prayer position at your heart. Inhale your arms out to the sides and overhead until your palms touch. Look up at your hands and arch your back slightly. Slowly exhale hands back down the center of your body to rest in front of your heart. Repeat this vinyasa in slow motion 5 times.

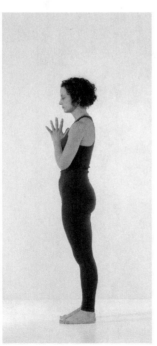
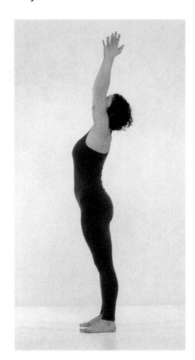
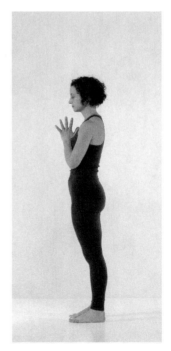

Vrksasana (Tree Pose)

Stand in Tadasana (Mountain Pose). Inhale and then exhale into your feet, feeling the support of the ground under them; repeat 3 times. On the fourth inhalation, lift your right leg up into Vrksasana. With your hands in prayer position at your heart, hold the pose for several slow, gentle breaths. As you exhale, lower your leg and change sides. Repeat again on both sides.

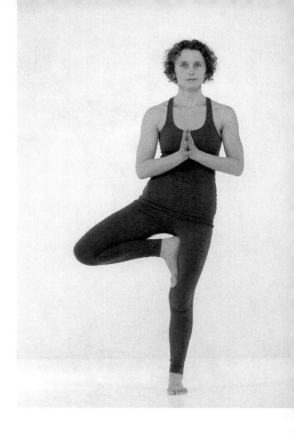

Ardha Chandrasana (Half-Moon Pose)

With your back against a wall, stand with your right foot parallel to and about 2 inches from the wall. Place a block about 6 inches in front of your right toes. Keeping your right foot where it is, bend your right knee, and place your hand on the block. Straighten your right leg as you lift your left leg up until it is parallel with the floor. Extend your left arm up toward the ceiling and either look up at your hand or straight ahead. Rest your torso, head, back, buttocks, leg, and arm against the wall. Rest here for as long as you like, breathing into your belly. Repeat on the other side.

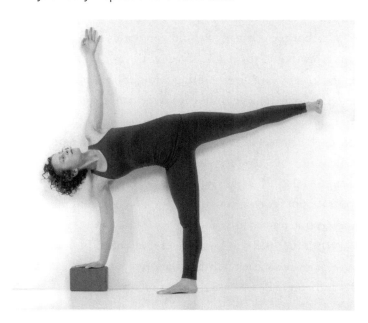

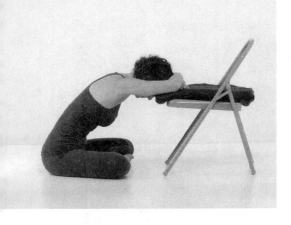

Sukhasana (Easy Seated Pose)

Sit in a comfortable cross-legged position with a chair in front of you, padded with a blanket. Inhale as you rise taller, then exhale as you bend forward and place your head in your arms on the chair. Breathe here, softly and naturally, for as long as you like. Recross your legs with the opposite leg in front and repeat the pose.

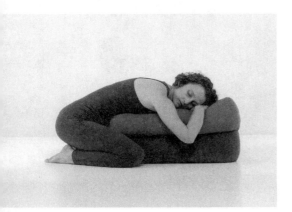

Supported Balasana (Child's Pose)

Sitting on your heels, spread your knees wider than your hips and bring your big toes together. Fold several blankets or stack two bolsters on top of each other; place them between your knees. Inhale as you lengthen your spine; exhale as you fold forward from your hips over your support. Lengthen the back of your neck, relax your shoulders, and cradle your head in your arms on your support. Stay here for several minutes or as long as you are comfortable.

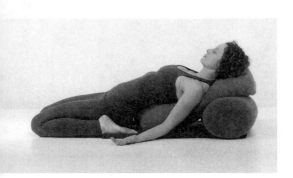

Supta Virasana (Reclining Hero Pose)

Place a bolster vertically behind you with another bolster underneath it to form a T. Kneel with your knees close together and your feet pointing straight back but wide enough apart for you to sit between them. Lean back on your forearms and gently let your torso and head rest on the bolsters. Close your eyes and breathe relaxing, nourishing breaths for as long as you like.

   BENEFITS: This pose is particularly good for lifting your diaphragm off your stomach, which should relieve indigestion and nausea and ease constipation.

   MODIFICATIONS: If your knees don't bend like this, sit on a block or lie back in Supta Baddha Konasana (Reclining Bound Angle Pose) with the soles of your feet together.

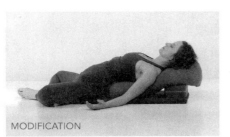

MODIFICATION

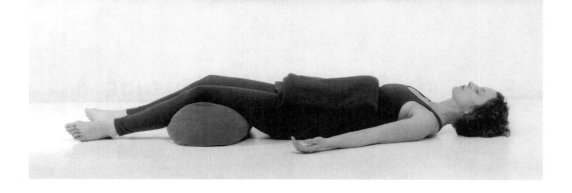

Savasana (Corpse Pose) with Hot Water Bottle

Lie on your back with your legs outstretched. If your back feels achy, position a bolster or rolled blanket under your knees. Place a hot water bottle (or heating pad on low to medium heat) on your belly with a folded blanket on top of that. Focus on your breathing, allowing it to bathe your belly with calm, healing energy. Stay here for at least 5 minutes. To come out, bend your knees, roll to your right side, and push yourself up with your arms.

FATIGUE

Even women who don't experience any other symptoms often find that fatigue sidelines them the first few months. In fact, fatigue may creep in before you even know you're pregnant because your body is already working overtime behind the scenes to make sure it can support you and your baby. The combination of increased blood production, soaring progesterone levels, low blood sugar, and low blood pressure may be enough to cause you to nod off in your dinner plate, according to Mayo Clinic. Having to get up several times a night to use the bathroom also contributes to not getting enough sleep. And sometimes, the anxiety you feel about your pregnancy—or the thought of becoming a mother—may be too much to bear without reaching for a blanket to pull over your head.

The most obvious way to combat fatigue is to give in to it. Rest when you can; go to sleep earlier than usual; sit outside in nature; and adjust your yoga practice to accommodate your energy level. Sometimes simply adding a few restorative or quieter poses to your usual practice is all you need to feel better. Other times, you'll want to do a shorter practice like Melissa's Fatigue Sequence to perk you up.

MELISSA'S FATIGUE SEQUENCE
MELISSA WILLIAMS

Feel free to link these poses together in a slow, sweet vinyasa, or simply choose those that work for you and linger in them as long as you wish.

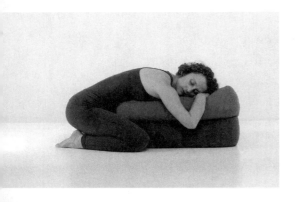

Balasana (Child's Pose)

Sitting on your heels, spread your knees wider than your hips and bring your big toes together. Fold several blankets or stack two bolsters on top of each other; place them between your knees. Inhale as you lengthen your spine; exhale as you fold forward from your hips over your support. Lengthen the back of your neck, relax your shoulders, and cradle your head in your arms on your support. Stay here for several minutes or as long as you are comfortable.

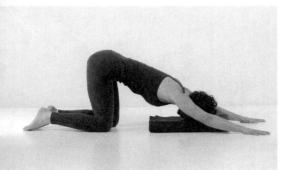

Uttana Shishosana (Extended Puppy Pose)

Start on your hands and knees. Fold one or two blankets on top of each other and place them in front of you. Keeping your hips stacked over your knees, stretch your arms forward into Shishosana. Inhale as you elongate your spine; exhale as you lengthen the back of your neck, relax your shoulders, and rest your head on your support. Stay here for several minutes or as long as you are comfortable.

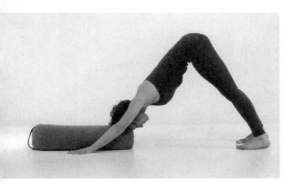

Adho Mukha Svanasana (Downward-Facing Dog Pose)

Come into Adho Mukha Svanasana, placing your feet wider apart than you usually would and bending your knees to help increase your circulation. Rest your head on a folded blanket, a block, or a bolster and remain here for several breaths, as long as you are comfortable.

Virabhadrasana II (Warrior II Pose)

From Tadasana (Mountain Pose) step your left foot back and come into Virabhadrasana II for 2 or 3 breaths. Then, on an inhalation, straighten your right knee and sweep your arms up overhead. As you exhale, bend the front knee again and extend the arms out from the shoulders, palms facing down. Moving in and out of the pose like this several times can help keep your breath long and smooth, focus your mind, and increase the circulation of life force throughout your body. Finish by holding Virabhadrasana II for 3 or 4 breaths. Repeat on the other side.

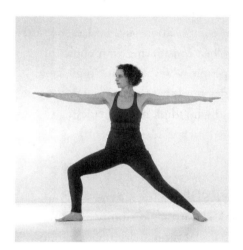 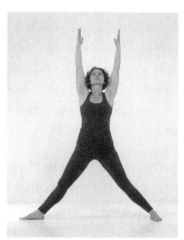 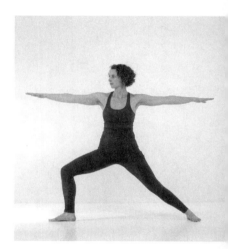

Utthita Trikonasana (Extended Triangle Pose)

Come into Utthita Trikonasana with your back against a wall. Using a block if necessary, extend your trunk, lift your chest and abdomen, and lean over your right leg. Rest your whole torso, the back of your head, and your arm against the wall. Remain in the pose for 3 to 5 breaths and then repeat on the other side.

NOTE: If you have time for only one pose, do Uttana Shishosana (Extended Puppy Pose) with your head supported on a folded blanket or a block.

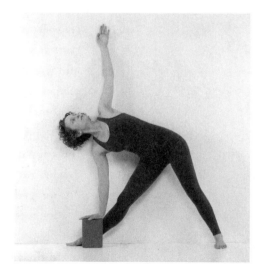

Getting Your Birthing Team Together

Some women prefer to see an OB/GYN soon after they discover they're pregnant; others would rather talk to a midwife first. Regardless of your choice, you'll want to assemble a prenatal team during your first trimester that includes both an OB/GYN and a midwife who will support your wishes for a safe, loving, and natural birthing experience. If you can, consider hiring both a midwife and a doula (birthing coach), because the two together may well increase your chances of birthing a healthier baby with no medical intervention. In fact, according to a 2013 Cochran Review of research studies released by the American College of Nurse-Midwives, women who used a midwife had fewer complications and far less medical intervention than those who did not. When considering your choice of midwife, doula, and OB/GYN, select people who share your yogic view of the body-mind connection, who understand that your emotions are just as important as your physical being, and who think of pregnancy as an exciting time of life and birthing as a natural and blessed event.

Coping with Miscarriage:
When the Unthinkable Happens

No woman wants to talk or even think about the possibility of losing her baby, but the sad truth is it happens. It's a lot more common than many people realize. Some statisticians say one out of five women suffer a miscarriage—others say one in ten; 85 percent of miscarriages happen in the first trimester. Risk factors exist (like smoking, alcohol and drug use, your age and your partner's age, infections, chronic diseases like type 2 diabetes, environmental toxins, and uterine abnormalities), as do reasons (like chromosomal abnormalities in about 70 percent of cases and improper placement of the egg in the placenta). But sometimes women who have none of the known risk factors lose their babies anyway, quite possibly because of an abnormality in the egg that rendered it nonviable. My friend Sara, who encouraged me to write this book, was one of those women. She miscarried at nine weeks, with no risk factors or problematic health history. She was young (only thirty-four) and healthy and had succeeded in giving birth naturally just three years earlier to a beautiful, healthy baby boy.

Sara already had a strong, established practice—she's practiced Ashtanga for more than ten years. She was careful to listen to her body, only doing what felt right, which allowed her to practice all through her first pregnancy and into her second one. While her yoga practice could not have prevented her miscarriage, it did help her heal from the trauma of losing her baby. By getting back on her mat, Sara could reconnect with her body and her heart and move from grief to gratitude.

NOTE: If you have a history of miscarriages or have had to be on bed rest to prevent one, you may want to shelve your regular practice and opt for more restorative, gentler poses until the end of your first trimester—just to be on the safe side.

Sara's Story

After my miscarriage, it took me about ten days of bleeding (and sobbing) to get back on my mat. By then I had stopped crying all the time and was beginning to feel like there might be life on the other side of the experience. Stepping onto the mat that evening was incredibly powerful. All my years of practice have taught me to come into myself as soon as I place my feet together at the top of my mat, big toes touching. Standing there with my eyes closed, my hands at my heart, I could see and feel everything so clearly: the incredible sense of loss that made my heart feel battered and bruised; the emptiness in my belly that just days before had been budding fullness and life. Tears started rolling down my cheeks, but I also felt the strength of my legs, my arms, and my core; the spaciousness of my mind; the collective heartbeat of the other people in the room and those beyond that. I moved through that practice with utter awareness. I cried on and off during my first Mysore practice after the loss, letting the waves of sadness and love move with me and my breath. This was the way to mourn the loss of my baby. This was the way to honor my baby's passing, to honor myself, and to connect with the pain and joy of all human beings throughout time. I have never been so grateful to be a practitioner of yoga.

ALLOWING YOUR PRACTICE TO SERVE YOU

As Sara discovered, getting back on your yoga mat after a miscarriage can often help you move through your grief. That practice may simply be lying in Savasana (Corpse Pose) or in a supported Supta Baddha Konasana (Reclining Bound Angle Pose) with your hands caressing your belly, sending thoughts of forgiveness and tender understanding to your womb. Other times, a slow vinyasa may ground your energy and allow you to remember your strength and welcome your vulnerability.

Here are some other strategies for getting through this rough time:

• Join a support group. Talking with other women who have been through similar experiences may help you let go of self-blame and feel less isolated.

• Share your grief with your partner. Even if your partner processes the loss of your baby in a different way, it doesn't mean that you can't both benefit from sharing your individual and collective pain.

• Let go of a timetable. Don't set a limit on how long to grieve. Yoga teaches us that feelings come and go on the wave of the breath, allowing us to feel whatever we feel deeply in the present moment. Some days may be more difficult than others, and that's okay.

• Try again—when you're ready. Most doctors recommend that you wait until you've had at least one predictable menstrual cycle (some even say three) before you get pregnant again for a couple reasons. First, your miscarriage may not actually be over. The residual tissue can cause a false positive on a pregnancy test and then, as it eventually works its way out of your body, the bleeding and cramping may give you the impression that you've miscarried again. Second, you'll have a hard time pinning down your last menstrual period, which doctors use to help establish the time of conception. This sounds like no big deal, but not knowing your due date can produce a lot of anxiety when you and your midwife or doctor are trying to chart the growth of your baby. Some women want to try again as soon as possible; others need a lot more time to prepare themselves physically and psychologically.

WELCOMING AND ACCEPTING: YOUR FIRST TRIMESTER PRACTICE

ELENA BROWER

This four-part practice (Recognize, Revisit, Remember, and Reset) can bring a sense of healing energy to your body and your nervous system, helping to create a healthy container in which your baby can grow and thrive. Your starting point—as in so many mindful practices—is simply an attentive, calm curiosity.

Set Your Intention

May this practice provide a spacious yet stabilizing experience for your first trimester. Use what feels good, start wherever you like, and marvel at every turn. Listen for what feels right to you; move the way your heart wants to move; and prepare your sacred, capable body to receive this life.

Invocation

Divine Mother, the Mother within, may I open myself fully to your guidance as my baby grows, as I surrender to my baby's birth, and as I walk the path that all mothers have walked before me.

RECOGNIZE

Take a comfortable seat on the floor and place your hands on either side of your belly. Set a timer for 10 minutes. Close your eyes and welcome your baby to his new home; let your whole body feel the gratitude and warmth of this welcome and reside in that sweet space as you watch your breath flow in and out of your lungs. Should your mind wander, gently return your attention to your belly and engage your baby once again.

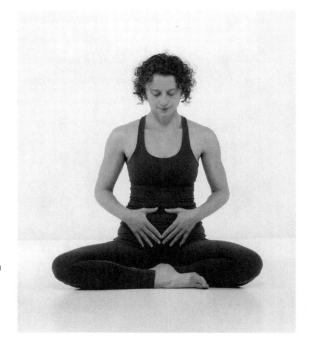

REVISIT

It's important to revisit your body often so you can create a healthy and joyous environment for your baby. Do this Revisit practice even if you only have a few minutes to spare, and see if you can experience a sweet flow of energy and perhaps a sense of inner balance. Maintain awareness of your natural breathing patterns throughout this practice, and time your movements to coincide with those patterns. Allow your body, riding the waves of your breath, to lead you home.

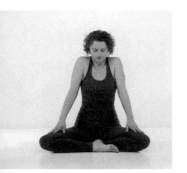 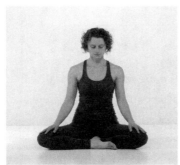

Shoulder Rolls

Begin in a comfortable cross-legged position. Keeping your gaze soft, inhale your shoulders up to your earlobes. Exhale them back, down, around, and forward. Do at least 11 circles, or keep going for as long as 3 minutes.

Sukhasana (Easy Seated Pose) Circles

Sitting in a cross-legged position, or in Sukhasana with your left shin in front of your right, place your hands on your thighs. Inhale as you round your spine. Exhale as you roll to one side, forward, and all the way around. Move through the rotation 7 times, then switch direction. Play with your breath, sending it into new places as you move.

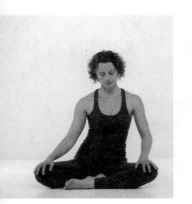 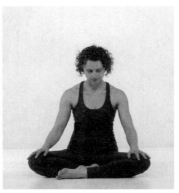 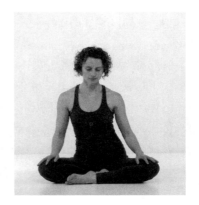 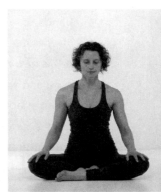

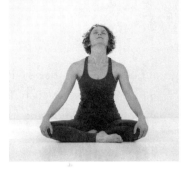
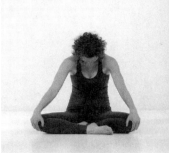

Marjaryasana to Bitilasana in Sukhasana (Cat/Cow in Easy Seated Pose)

Remaining in Sukhasana, switch your leg position (right shin in front of your left) and place your hands on your knees. Inhale as you arch your back and look up, keeping your chest broad. Exhale as you round your back, look down and in. Play with the tempo, moving quickly when that feels good and then slowly, thoughtfully, and deliberately. Do what feels good today. Repeat 6 or 7 times—opening and closing—and then make your way up to standing.

Tadasana (Mountain Pose) with Circle Variations

Stand tall in Tadasana. With your hands on your waist, make huge circles with your hips, 7 times in one direction and then 7 in the other. Make the movements big and let your breath really dictate the rhythm of the rotations.

Come back to Tadasana. Extend your right leg straight out in front of you and lift it off the floor. Shake out that leg by making circles at the ankle. Bring your right foot back to the floor and reverse sides. Do each leg circle several times.

Now extend your right arm and shake it out all the way to your fingertips a few times; release any physical discomfort—and any doubt or emotional pain you feel in your heart—out and down through that arm and past your

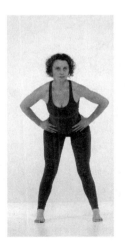
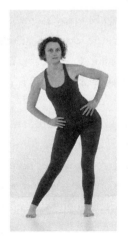
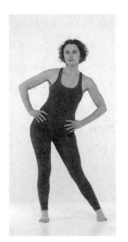
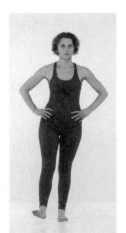
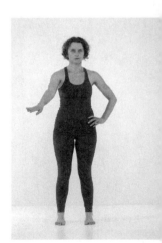

fingertips. Shake it away until it feels better. Then rotate your hand at your wrist a few times in each direction. Drop your right arm down to your side and repeat the movements with your left arm.

REMEMBER

Begin this part of the practice with Surya Namaskars (Sun Salutations) to warm up, modifying as you go if anything doesn't feel good or if you feel tired or nauseous. If you've had challenges conceiving, you may want to focus on rest and meditation. Allow your body to receive the new life and don't try to move, push, or prove anything. If you're ready to move, have fun with this sequence, make it your own, and revel in the wonders of your body.

Surya Namaskar (Sun Salutation)

Stand tall in Tadasana (Mountain Pose) with your feet parallel and slightly wider apart than usual. Keeping your legs strong, inhale your arms over your head in Urdhva Hastasana (Upward Salute). Exhale as you fold over your legs into Uttanasana (Standing Forward Bend), remaining there as long as you like. Relax your toes, and breathe deeply.

Whenever you're ready, inhale into the back of your belly to extend your heart forward as you lift up into Ardha Uttanasana (Half Standing Forward Bend), with your hands on your shins. On your next exhalation, put your hands back on your mat and step back into Phalakasana (Plank Pose), with your knees either lifted or on the floor. Slowly lower yourself to the floor, and inhale your heart forward into either Bhujangasana (Cobra Pose) or Urdhva Mukha Svanasana (Upward-Facing Dog Pose). Exhale back up to Adho Mukha Svanasana (Downward-Facing Dog Pose). Take a few breaths here, with particular emphasis on opening and breathing into the back of your belly, "behind" your baby.

On an exhalation, soften your knees, look forward, and walk your feet toward the front of your mat to stand in Uttanasana. With your legs strong, inhale your arms up overhead, and then exhale your hands down to prayer position at your heart. Close your eyes and take a moment to focus on your baby and the sacred space you've made for her. Repeat this sequence 3 to 4 times.

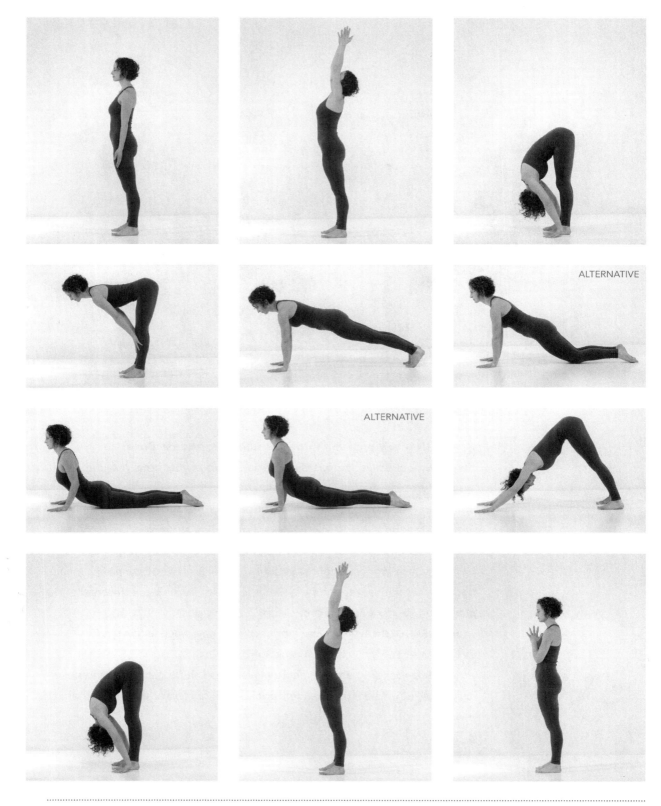

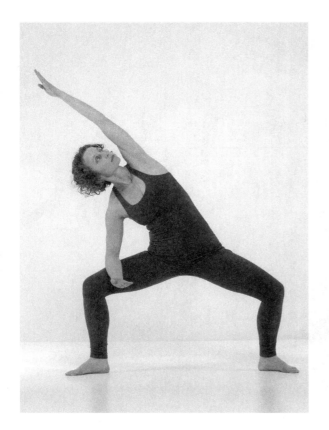
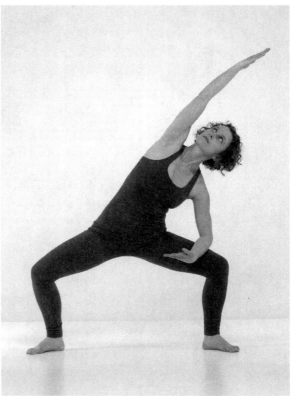

Parsva Utkata Konasana (Side-Stretching Goddess Pose)

Step your feet as far apart as is comfortable, open your arms out to the sides at shoulder height, bend your knees, and lean to your right, placing your right elbow on your right knee. Stretch your left arm over your head, and breathe the left side of your body wide open—from your waist to between your ribs and all the way up under your arm. Stay here and breathe space into your right side until you feel a sense of symmetry. Inhale back to center, then repeat the pose to your left. Inhale back to center, straighten your knees, and prepare for standing poses.

MODIFICATIONS: If you feel fatigued, you may practice this side-stretching sequence with your back against a wall.

NOTE: Depending on your energy level, you can do each standing pose separately (right side and then left side) or string a few of them together in a vinyasa.

Virabhadrasana II (Warrior II)

Standing with your feet as wide apart as is comfortable, turn your right foot out to 90 degrees and your left foot in slightly. Bend your right knee and come into Virabhadrasana II. Feel the strength of your legs as they connect to the earth, allowing your arms and upper body to feel light, open, and soft. Breathe here for 3 to 5 breaths, listening with reverence to what your body needs. Repeat on the left side.

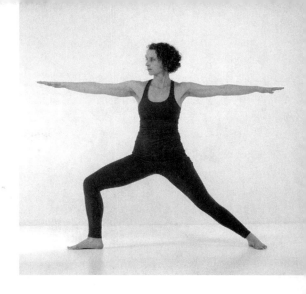

Utthita Parsvakonasana (Extended Side-Angle Pose)

Return to Virabhadrasana II (Warrior II) on the right side. As you exhale, place your right elbow on your right knee and begin to turn your belly, ribs, and chest up toward the ceiling, coming into a slight backbend. Stretch your left arm over your head, and breathe here for several breaths. Return through Virabhadrasana II and repeat on the left side. End in Virabhadrasana II.

BENEFITS: This pose offers strength and stability coupled with flexibility and receptivity.

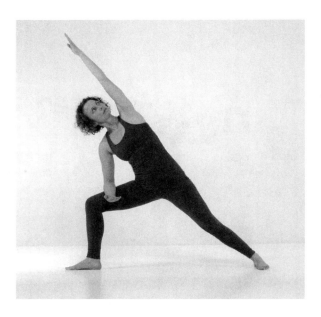
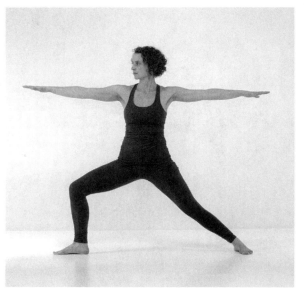

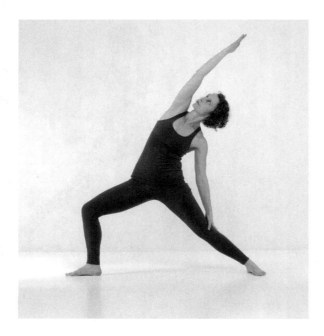

Viparita Virabhadrasana (Reverse Warrior Pose)

From Virabhadrasana II (Warrior II Pose), keep the front knee bent and move your back hand down the outside back thigh. Inhale your front arm straight up toward the ceiling, keeping your bicep close to your ear. Hold for 3 breaths, then either move into Ardha Chandrasana (Half-Moon Pose) or repeat this pose on the other side.

Ardha Chandrasana (Half-Moon Pose)

From Warrior II, place a block in front of and just outside your front foot, close up your stance, and move into Ardha Chandrasana. Lift up and flex the back foot as you inhale. Keep your hand on your waist or extend your arm up toward the ceiling. Relax your throat, jaw, and eyes. Soften your belly and release any holding in the groin and pelvic floor. Stay here for several breaths, and then slowly come out of the pose, returning for a breath into Warrior II Pose. Repeat on the other side or move on to the next pose.

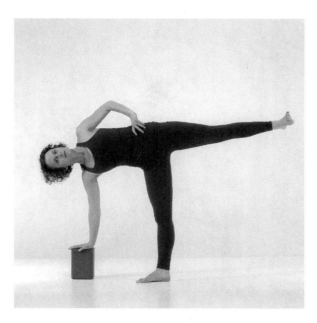

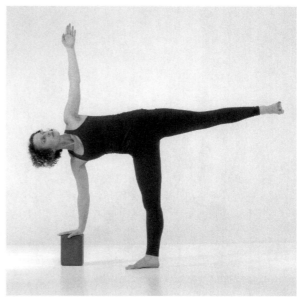

Utthita Trikonasana (Extended Triangle Pose)

From Virabhadrasana II (Warrior 2 Pose), straighten your right leg, and keeping your weight evenly distributed in both feet, come into Utthita Trikonasana. Feel the strength of your legs as they connect to the earth, allowing your arms and upper body to feel light, open, and soft. Remain here for 3 to 5 breaths. Repeat on the other side or move to the next pose.

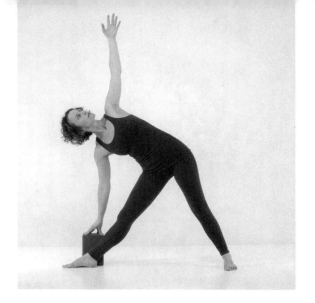

Parsvottansana (Intense Side Stretch)

From Utthita Trikonasana (Extended Triangle Pose), close up your stance about halfway. Turn toward your front leg, look up at the ceiling, and then, keeping both legs strong and straight, bend over your front leg, resting your hands on the floor (or on blocks). Release your head and neck down toward your shin. If you feel dizzy or your balance is a little off, keep your head up. Breathe here for a few breaths, and either repeat on the other side or move into Uttanasana (Standing Forward Bend).

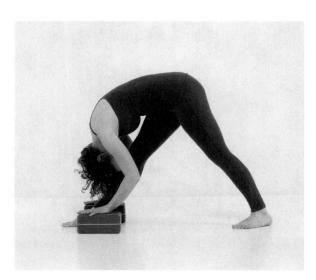

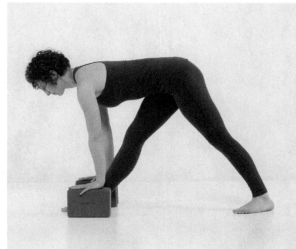

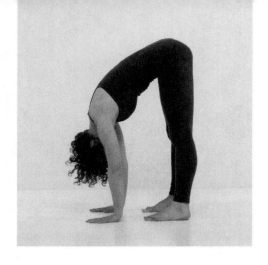

Uttanasana (Standing Forward Bend)

From Parsvottanasana (Intense Side Stretch), bring your back leg forward so your feet are at least hip-width apart. Keep your hands on the floor (or on blocks) out in front of your feet. Remain here for several breaths, then bend both knees and slowly step back into Adho Mukha Svanasana (Downward-Facing Dog Pose).

Adho Mukha Svanasana (Downward-Facing Dog Pose)

Rooting your hands firmly into the mat, press back into Adho Mukha Svanasana. If you feel tired or nauseous, move into Balasana (Child's Pose) or Uttana Shishosana (Extended Puppy Pose) instead.

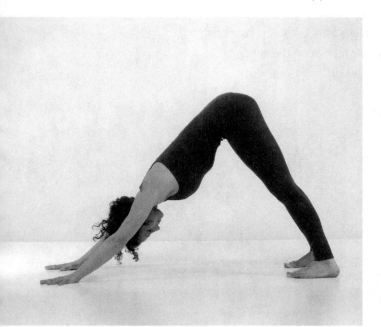

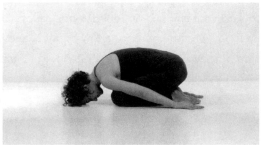

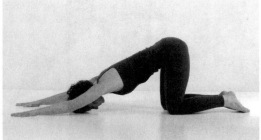

Malasana (Garland Pose)

From Adho Mukha Svanasana (Downward-Facing Dog Pose), exhale your right foot forward to the outside of and behind your right hand. inhale; exhale your left leg forward to the outside of and behind your left hand. Come into a squat. You can sit on a block (or rest your back against the wall) if that's more comfortable today. Lengthen your arms and release your head and neck. Move your left hand to the outside of your left foot and, raising your right arm, twist to the right. Exhale and repeat the twist to the left. Come back to center and slowly move into a seated position for the next pose.

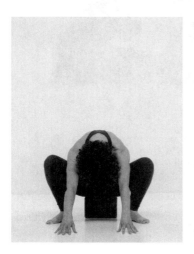 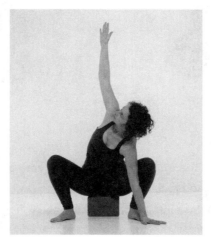 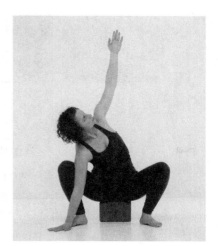

Baddha Konasana (Bound Angle Pose)

Sitting upright (on a cushion or a block if necessary to release your pelvis forward), bend your knees and place the soles of your feet together, allowing your knees to fall to the sides. For a more relaxed, comfortable pose, place a rolled blanket or a block under each thigh to support your legs. Remain in this pose for several breaths or as long as you wish.

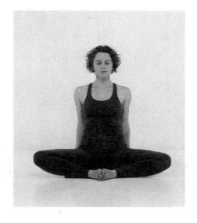 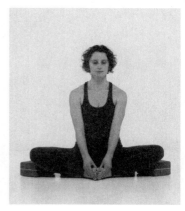

Paschimottanasana (Seated Forward Bend)

Sit with your legs straight out in front of you, a little more than hip-width apart. Extend forward from your hips, then release your back, head, and neck toward your shins. For a more restful pose, place two folded blankets or a bolster on your outstretched legs, and rest your torso and head on your support. Remain here for several breaths.

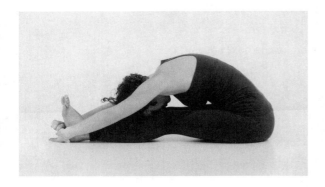

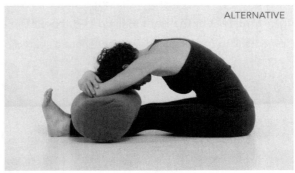

ALTERNATIVE

Rest

Perhaps the most important part of your practice is the time you take to absorb and receive the opening, the revitalized circulation, and the healing. During this time, I found that simply resting my own hands on my belly and heart helped me cultivate receptivity and gave me the opportunity to really listen to my body.

Lie down in Savasana (Corpse Pose). Notice the quality of your breath as it flows through your lungs. Is one lung more receptive than the other? Does one side of your body feel more open than the other? Take this time to cultivate symmetry in your breathing, and let your thoughts rest in the center of your torso, in and around your heart.

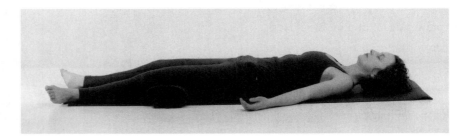

Take the last few minutes to rest your hands on either side of your belly, and breathe into that space until your body feels softer and quieter. Simply enjoy being on your back while you still can!

Reset

Use this practice to become familiar with what's going on inside and find a level of comfort in your own skin. Doing this just a few moments every day may give you more ease in your thinking. Come to a comfortable seated position like Sukhasana (Easy Seated Pose), close your eyes, and listen deeply, noticing the trains of thought looping around your brain. Simply sit, breathe, and observe the thoughts as they arise. Notice them without latching on, and see if you can put a little more space between them, using your conscious breath and presence to slow them down. Consider yourself a researcher. Observe. Slow down.

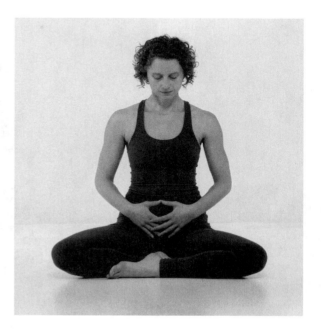

Pranayama Modifications for the First Trimester

During your first trimester, focus on pranayama practices that balance your emotions, especially when you feel anxious, scared, or weepy; those that balance your energy, especially if you're fatigued or agitated; and those that expand your lung capacity. Steer clear of any breathing exercises in which you retain the breath either after the inhalation (Antara Kumbhaka) or after the exhalation (Bahya Kumbhaka). Stop any pranayama if you get light-headed or start hyperventilating and return to your regular breath pattern.

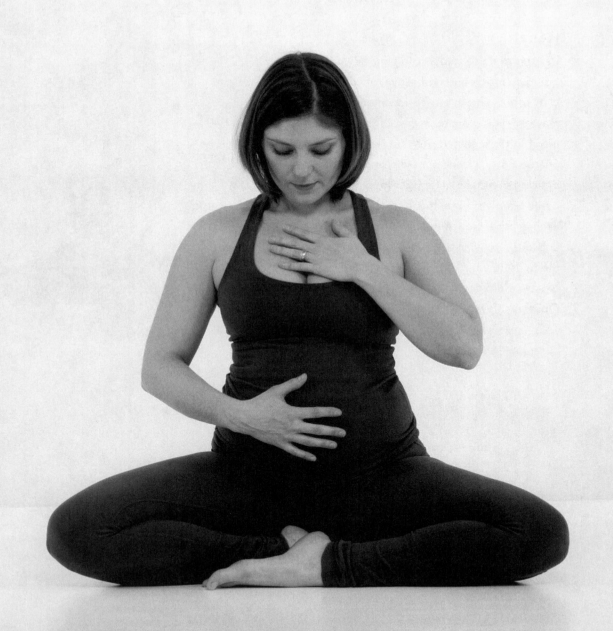

2.

SECOND TRIMESTER

Rooting Down and Looking Within
From Fourteen to Twenty-Seven Weeks

Sequences by Stephanie Snyder
and Melissa Williams

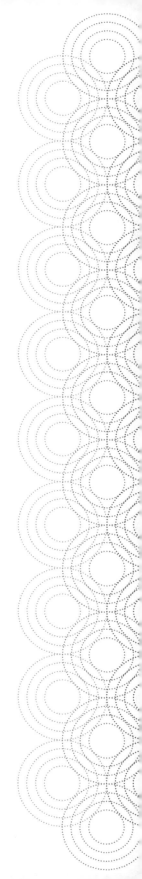

As you begin the transition from the often-wobbly uncertainty of the first trimester to the relative stability of the second, you're probably starting to feel a bit more confident, a tad less queasy, and a lot more eager to get back to your yoga practice if you've taken a break. Those first three months can be overwhelming (especially for first-time moms) and sometimes anxiety producing. According to the typical Western process, you've no doubt been poked, prodded, blood tested, ultrasounded, and lectured on what could go wrong, as though your pregnancy were a disease to manage instead of an occasion to celebrate. For the most part, this trimester is blessedly devoid of such intrusions, and you'll probably have more energy, so enjoy the time you have to connect more deeply with your baby and trust in your ability to birth him in the most natural and loving way.

But how do you trust yourself if you don't know what to think or whom to believe? Yoga can help by providing a firm foundation from which to begin and a sense of direction. In other words, you need to know where you are before you can know where you're going. Pregnancy catapults you into the unknown, and if you come into the second trimester without an anchor, you can too easily get buffeted by the voices and opinions of doctors, well-meaning friends, relatives, and even perfect strangers, at the expense of your own intuition.

The focus for your practice right now becomes rooting down and looking within, resting your mind in a calm, unbroken flow of attention—the definition of *abhyasa*—so you can truly know yourself. This self-understanding will help you, now and throughout your pregnancy, to choose actions and advice that move you toward the most healthful and positive outcome for you and your baby. At the same time, practicing *vairagya* (detachment) will encourage you to set aside those things that stand in your way and ultimately be okay with whatever experiences you end up having.

Reenergize Your Practice

If you've practiced all through the first trimester, you can continue doing what you've been doing, with some allowances for your growing belly. If you've had to table your practice in favor of saltines and ginger tea, you will likely be able to return to your pre-pregnancy practice without a problem. From here on, you'll benefit more from yoga by shifting your attention inward, listening to what you and your baby need, and responding accordingly. By the fifth month, your ability to listen may get a lot easier because you'll actually be able to see changes in your body and maybe feel your baby move. Practicing yoga with love and devotion— what yogis call *sraddha*—can help you trust your body and your intuition. Embracing the full spectrum of asana and pranayama will prepare you for the months ahead and give you the strength and confidence to birth your baby.

At the beginning of this trimester, depending on your energy level (and how quickly your belly bump emerges), your practice can remain pretty much the same as it's always been, so long as it still feels good. While you certainly want to get the most out of your practice, you also want to minimize any risk to your baby. So in the latter part of the trimester, twenty-five to twenty-seven weeks, you'll need to either cut out some poses completely or change the way you do them to accommodate your expanding belly, your fatigue levels, and your emotional health. Here are some important questions to ask yourself during your practice now:

- Does this pose (or sequence) create more space in my body or less?
- Does it expand my abdomen or compress it?
- Does it bring more breath into my abdomen or make breathing more difficult?
- Am I comfortable in this position? Is my baby?

Choose poses for their ability to open up the front of your body, create space for your baby to move and grow, and elongate your spine. If you have favorite, must-do poses, modify them so they can accomplish these things too.

Making Modifications

No matter what style of yoga you practiced before you got pregnant, most teachers agree on a few essential modifications to protect the baby and keep you healthy. Before getting into specific modifications, though, it's worth mentioning a few general practice caveats.

First and foremost, if you start bleeding or experience any unusual cramping, stop your practice and immediately call your doctor. Second, if you still get waves of prenatal nausea, don't soldier on. Slow way down when the queasiness hits or go back to doing My Morning Sickness Sequence on page 16. And third, if you've always done a physically challenging practice but find your belly is getting in the way, scale back a notch or two.

Other modifications are more specific, but they're all pretty commonsensical, and they focus on a central theme: make your baby as comfortable as possible. For example, if you love a strong power yoga practice in a heated room, lower the thermostat, open a window, and dial back the intensity. Why? Because if you're sweating, your baby's overheated, and that's dangerous. Studies show that prolonged exposure to high temperatures can cause hyperthermia in the mother and neural tube defects in the fetus. That's why saunas or hot tubs (over 100°F) are also off-limits when you're pregnant. Don't risk taking a sixty- or ninety-minute hot yoga class when practicing in a cooler, well-ventilated room is a safer option.

Most styles of yoga have their own dos and don'ts, but they all agree that you shouldn't compress your belly or cut off circulation to your uterus and that you should practice with mindful attention and loving awareness of your growing baby.

IYENGAR

Although most practitioners use props these days, Iyengar teachers have mastered the fine art of supported yoga. Using blocks, bolsters, and straps, or doing poses at the wall, allows you to reap the benefits of practice all through your pregnancy. In her book *Yoga: A Gem for Women*, Geeta Iyengar encourages women to keep doing yoga, with some modifications, as long as the practice itself isn't tiring. She says you should experience a "feeling of radiant health after you practice." If you feel fatigued or exhausted instead, either the practice isn't the right one for you at that moment or you have overdone it. "It is wrong to overstrain," Iyengar says. Her advice includes stepping (not jumping) your legs apart in standing poses; extending through your spine rather than bending forward in seated forward bends, keeping your back slightly concave and your chest lifted so your baby has room to move; and not practicing inversions like Sirsasana (Headstand) and Sarvangasana (Shoulderstand) unless you've done them in your pre-pregnancy life.

ASHTANGA

Unless you're one of those practitioners who can effortlessly float to the top of your mat or glide seamlessly into Chaturanga—with a prominent belly leading the way—your Ashtanga or vinyasa teacher will probably advise you to skip the jump backs and jump throughs; they can be too jarring for the fetus, and you can too easily lose your balance. Stepping back or stepping through into a wider stance than usual works just as well. Like Geeta Iyengar, Pattabhi Jois encouraged women to keep their chest extended and to place their hands out in front of their feet during forward bends.

VINYASA

Vinyasa practitioners—no matter what particular style they prefer—can't imagine doing yoga without some form of Surya Namaskars, which are perfectly fine throughout most of your pregnancy. By the time you're really showing though (which can be as early as fifteen weeks or as late as twenty-five weeks), you'll want to adjust some aspects of those Sun Salutations. Again, modify with these rules in mind: don't squish the baby, don't compromise your ability to breathe, and don't put pressure on your pubic bones by spreading your legs too wide in standing poses like Virabhadrasana (Warrior Pose) or Utthita Trikonasana (Triangle Pose) or in wide-legged seated poses. Too much pressure can cause the bones to sheer, which hurts. Do widen your stance in closed-legged standing poses and forward bends—remember the focus is on making space. Instead of bending forward, lift and extend your spine forward. Be mindful of your balance—as your belly protrudes, your center of gravity shifts. And let the rhythm and quality of your breathing determine the intensity of your practice.

Stephanie Snyder, the vinyasa teacher who created the sequence on page 63, always recommends that her pregnant students place their hands on blocks when doing standing forward bends, even if they can still touch the floor with ease, to help them extend their spine. This also helps keep the chest open, the head up, the collarbones wide, and the side body lifted. Extending instead of rounding the spine gives you the additional benefit of containing the stretch, which helps stabilize your sacrum—always an at-risk area during pregnancy because of the hormone relaxin—and prevent sacroiliac pain, a common complaint for women in the second trimester.

NOTE: No matter which trimester you're in, give up or modify any poses that don't feel good to you for any reason, poses that cause dizziness or shortness of breath, or any form of pranayama that requires you to hold your breath.

By the time you're well into your second trimester (twenty-four to twenty-seven weeks), you can pretty much forget about lying flat on your belly. Why? Experts say that being on your belly (or even bending forward in seated forward bends with your legs close together) can compress the blood vessels and nerves in your uterus. However, lying on your back, once you start to show, isn't a good idea either. The weight of your uterus can bear down on and compress the vena cava—a major blood vessel located to the right of your spine. The vena cava delivers blood to your baby, and constricting it can put her at risk and leave you feeling dizzy, short of breath, and nauseous.

Practicing Prenatal Yoga

Many women turn to yoga for the first time when they're pregnant, urged on by their midwife or OB/GYN. So naturally a lot of experienced yoga practitioners shy away from prenatal classes, assuming they'll be too beginner-focused or too restorative, and these women couldn't imagine lying over a bolster for the next six months. In fact, their assumptions are inaccurate. Prenatal yoga is almost as diverse as other styles of yoga—Ashtanga, Iyengar, Kripalu, kundalini, vinyasa, power yoga—because it springs from those traditions. Adding a weekly prenatal class to your normal routine makes a lot of sense, not least because practicing with other pregnant women can help you resist doing poses that might not suit your body. And since women can benefit from being with other women who are at different stages of pregnancy, you'll have the opportunity to learn from others' experiences and to share your own.

Jane Austin, a prenatal teacher and childbirth educator in San Francisco, feels that prenatal yoga prepares women to give birth, no matter what trimester they're in. "The yoga postures are definitely designed to strengthen the body," she says. But equally important, they help create suppleness in a woman's body "so she can open when the time comes to birth her baby." The prenatal pranayama practices also support the work of labor because they show women how to use the breath as a means of opening. According to Jane, "Birthing a baby requires great effort but also the ability to completely let go. We cultivate this in our yoga practice so that we can take it off the mat and into labor and birth."

When we think of support in yoga, we often picture a closet or shelf full of props. But support also comes in the form of community, which is another thing that a prenatal class provides. Chances are the women in your class will understand what you're going through. Reach out to them. Toward the end of the second trimester, a surprising level of anxiety and fear can sometimes arise. Janice Gates, a long-time yoga teacher from Marin County, says when that happens, we often think we need to relax, take warm baths, or lie down and pull the blankets over our head until the feelings subside. What we need instead is a sense of direction; we need to take action. The antidote for anxiety is not restorative yoga; lying still may just amplify the mind's chatter. In these situations, you need to get moving and shift your attention out of your head and into your feet. Once you've moved your body, you can ease into a guided meditation practice like Yoga Nidra (Yoga Sleep), or a long, sweet Savasana.

Jaclyn's Story

Jaclyn Roberson, a long-time yoga student, signed up for a prenatal class when she was four months along, even though she continued to enjoy her regular Ashtanga classes. "When I was finally able to take a prenatal class at sixteen weeks," she says, "it was a breath of fresh air." As a dedicated runner, she discovered that prenatal yoga allowed her to let go of her ego and find more space in her practice, performing fewer poses, and even using props. She had never really used props before, but she says, "By allowing myself to be supported, I learned to love and respect my body on a new level." As her pregnancy progressed, Jaclyn loved being able to share her experiences and concerns with other like-minded pregnant mothers in the class.

The Inside Scoop

What is actually happening in your womb during these three months? Plenty, as it turns out—most of which you remain blissfully unaware. Of course, it's all about the baby's needs, and the body's only too happy to rise to the occasion and fulfill those needs. The hormones are still raging, even though your hCG levels have dropped—which means no more nausea, or at least not as much. The placenta churns out loads of extra fluid, which accounts for about half the weight you'll gain now. This fluid circulates through the bloodstream, softening your joints and ligaments to give your baby more room and preparing your tissues, muscles, and organs for labor and birthing. All this softening, however, can sometimes make your joints a little too loosey-goosey, so be careful not to move too deeply into your squats or stretch your muscles too much. Your body pumps up the volume—of blood, that is—to about 40 percent more than normal by the end of the second trimester, and it relaxes the blood vessel walls so they can more easily deliver oxygen and nutrients to the baby. To carry all that extra fluid, your blood pressure decreases, which might make you feel dizzy if you lift your head out of a pose too quickly. And since your baby's going to need additional fat from you by the end of your pregnancy, your body begins to stockpile it more efficiently. With all this relaxation going on in your blood vessels, don't be surprised if your gums bleed more readily, you end up with varicose veins or hemorrhoids, or (this one's more fun) your sex drive revs up.

While all that's taking place behind the scenes, a lot is happening on the main stage too. Front and center, so to speak, your breasts have already gotten bigger (as the milk ducts swell in preparation for lactation), and your belly has started to expand to give the baby more room. In fact, you may already be showing by the fourth or fifth month (especially if you're having your second or third baby).

The baby's sex organs have already formed, so an ultrasound can now determine whether you have a boy or a girl incubating, should you decide to find out. She has hair on her head and teeny tiny eyebrows and lashes, and her ribs and spine have hardened. These three months are a time for growth—for you and your baby—more than development.

Around week 20, if you stay very quiet, close your eyes, and place your hands on your belly, you may be able to feel the first flutters of life. Of course soon enough (by week 25 or so), those gentle butterfly kisses will turn into pokes, jabs, and kicks. While you're busy admiring your baby's somersault performance, he's listening to the sound of your voice and moving to the music you play. In fact, according to a few recent studies, he's been privy to your conversations and musical tastes since week 16, quite a bit earlier than researchers first thought. Interestingly enough, he's listening and responding, even before his ears are completely developed. Several studies suggest that a mother's stress level during pregnancy can impact her baby both in the womb, where one study says he appears to have a harder time tuning out outside stimuli, and after he's born, when he can show signs of depression and irritability.

Ayurvedic healers say you should take care in choosing which movies you watch and even what books you read, since your baby will not only hear your words but can detect and be affected by your emotions as well. As the ayurvedic expert Dr. Welch puts it, the "grooves of the mother's mind affect the baby's heart."

So talk to your baby, sing, laugh, play music. Such joyful activities may very well up his postnatal happiness quotient. Equally important, design your yoga practice to keep your own anxiety levels in check as much as you can. Adding quiet, harmonious music to your yoga practice, at least during Savasana, may help calm your nerves and reassure your baby. As Curt Sandman, one of the authors of a 2011 study published in *Psychological Science* journal, says, "We believe that the human fetus is collecting information for life after birth; it's preparing for life based on messages the mom is providing."

An Interactive Savasana (Corpse Pose)

Take two bolsters (or two thick folded blankets) and place them behind you in a T formation—the one on the bottom parallel to the wall and the one on top perpendicular. Sit in front of them with your sacrum on the floor and your legs outstretched. Lie back so that your torso and head are resting on the top bolster; you can use a pillow if you wish. In this completely relaxed state, rub a generous amount of warmed almond, jojoba, or unrefined sesame oil on your hands. As you slowly and lovingly massage your belly, matching your breath to your movements, sing, chant, or talk to your baby. Then relax even more deeply in silence for as long as you wish. Repeat this activity as often as possible.

Second Trimester Challenges

Entering your second trimester doesn't necessarily mean you'll suddenly suffer from heartburn, hip pain, bleeding gums, constipation, and hemorrhoids, but hormonal surges make these symptoms more likely now than in your pre-pregnancy life. Relaxin, the hormone responsible for the uterine muscles softening to accommodate a growing baby, doesn't confine its services to the pelvic area. This hormone relaxes *all* smooth muscle tissue, including the digestive tract, which can increase indigestion, gastric distress, and constipation.

If you have hip pain that radiates down your leg, it may feel like sciatica, but it's more likely you have a condition called pelvic girdle pain. Guess what? You can blame relaxin for this too, because it can cause instability in the joints. Eric Franklin, creator of the Franklin Method, explains in his book *Pelvic Power* that this instability can cause one side of the pelvis to move more than the other side, which can irritate the joints and ligaments. Just like sciatica, the pain usually happens on one side (it can even change sides sometimes), and it may run down the back of your leg. You'll probably feel it most acutely in your buttocks or hips or around your sacroiliac joints. Doing the pelvic floor exercises in Chapter 3 can help you create more stability in your pelvis and hopefully find some relief.

All the excess hormones and the increase in bodily fluids that disrupted your sleep in the first trimester—causing you to get up several times each night to pee—have subsided somewhat now. But something else equally annoying has taken their place: finding a position comfortable enough to let you sleep through the night. My daughter Megan stopped sleeping on her stomach by the time she was four months into her pregnancy. Not because she might endanger her baby, but psychologically, she said she just didn't feel comfortable. She kept thinking she was squishing him! At twenty weeks, even though she was barely showing, she couldn't sleep on her back either. "Whenever I was on my back too long, I felt a lot of pressure on my diaphragm," she says. She wasn't feeling the baby's weight or position yet, but the weight of her expanding uterus made it difficult for her to breathe. Megan had to train herself to sleep on her left side, which wasn't easy for her.

As I mentioned earlier, once your belly has expanded, lying flat on your back is not a good idea because the weight of your uterus against the vena cava (the main blood supply to the placenta) can reduce the blood flow to your baby, delivering less oxygen and fewer nutrients. It can also cause hemorrhoids, fluctuations in your own blood pressure, and muscle pain. Since the vena cava is on the right side of your spine, lying on your left side is preferable, but don't worry if you fall asleep on your right side. The most important thing is not to lie completely flat on your back all night long. That probably won't happen, though. As Megan pointed out, lying flat makes it too hard to breathe.

Sound (Sleep) Advice

Kathryn Templeton, ayurvedic expert

By the time the second trimester rolls around, your ability to sleep may become doubly compromised. Your racing mind (from excitement as much as anxiety) makes it hard to settle in for the night, and finding a position you're comfortable with can make sleep a choreographed ballet of pillow shifts whenever you want to turn over. Try these suggestions to calm your mind and at least minimize the tossing and turning:

- Turn off the TV at least an hour before bed.
- During this time, resist online anything—shopping, Twitter, Facebook, news gathering, or working.
- Use that extra hour for self-reflection, journal writing, restorative yoga, or meditation.
- Treat yourself to a warm bath followed by a foot massage with lavender-scented sesame oil.
- Make yourself some warm almond milk sprinkled with sleep-inducing herbs, such as cinnamon, cardamom, nutmeg, and saffron, and a teaspoon of ghee.
- Earlier in the day, preferably no later than 4 P.M., practice Yoga Nidra (Yoga Sleep). If you practice this too close to bedtime, it may refresh your energy instead of moving you into sleep.

While yoga can't reduce the number of trips you take to the bathroom, it can help ease your indigestion and hip pain—and even help you get some rest. The short sequences that follow may help by creating space between your digestive organs and your baby and by releasing tightness in your joints. If you only have time for one pose, look at the end of each sequence for Melissa's recommendation.

MELISSA'S SEQUENCE FOR INDIGESTION
MELISSA WILLIAMS

Poses that lift your diaphragm away from your expanding uterus may relieve your heartburn. Try any or all of these poses to see what works for you.

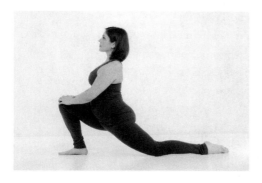

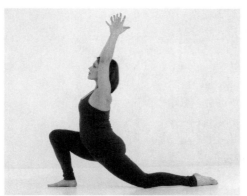

Anjaneyasana (Low Lunge Pose)
Start in Adho Mukha Svanasana (Downward-Facing Dog Pose) or on your hands and knees. Exhale your right foot forward between your hands and drop your left knee down into a low lunge. You can scoot your left knee away from your hips until you feel a gentle stretch in the front of your left thigh and groin. Bring both hands to your front knee and lift your torso up and away from your waist. You may extend your arms overhead, if you wish. Hold here for 3 breaths, then exhale your torso over your front thigh and return to your starting position before switching sides.

BENEFITS: This pose helps relieve indigestion by lifting the weight of the baby off your digestive organs.

Supta Baddha Konasana
(Reclining Bound Angle Pose)

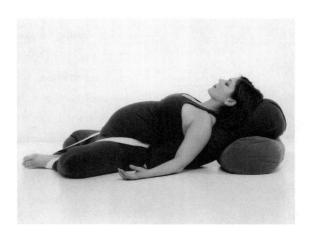

Place two bolsters behind you to form a T, with the vertical bolster on top on a slant from top to bottom. Slip a loosely buckled strap over your head and move it down to your sacrum. Loop the strap under your feet so that it stretches over your ankles and rests on the tops of your thighs. Now lie back so that your whole torso and head rest comfortably on the top bolster and your buttocks and legs are on the mat. Cinch the belt securely. Close your eyes and rest in this pose for as long as you like, breathing deeply and smoothly.

MODIFICATIONS: If you feel any strain in your neck, support it with a folded blanket positioned on the top bolster. To ease any discomfort in your lower back, move away from the bolsters slightly.

BENEFITS: This restorative pose lifts your diaphragm off your stomach, which should help alleviate most digestive disorders. It also broadens your pelvis, releases any tension in your back, and makes more space for your baby.

Balasana (Child's Pose)

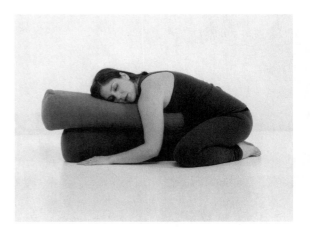

Place two bolsters (or a few folded blankets) in front of you, one on top of the other. Sit with your knees wide to accommodate the bolsters and your belly and with your big toes close together. Keeping your sacrum close to your heels, bend forward onto the bolsters so that your upper torso and head are resting on them and your belly is between your knees. Lengthen the back of your neck, close your eyes, and relax your head and arms. Remain in this pose for as long as you like.

BENEFITS: This pose calms your central nervous system and fires up the heat (*agni*) in your belly that aids digestion. Added benefits include the release of tension in your hip joints, groin, and pelvic floor muscles.

Side-Lying Savasana

Lying on your left side, straighten your left leg. Bend your right leg and place the knee, shin, and foot on a bolster that you've positioned in front of and parallel to your straight left leg. (Don't put the bolster between your legs; only under the top, bent knee.) Rest your head and arm on a bolster or folded blanket so that it's in line with your spine. Remain in the pose for as long as you like, at least 3 to 5 minutes.

BENEFITS: This pose helps your kidneys process and eliminate excess waste and fluids; balances your nervous system, and relieves anxiety.

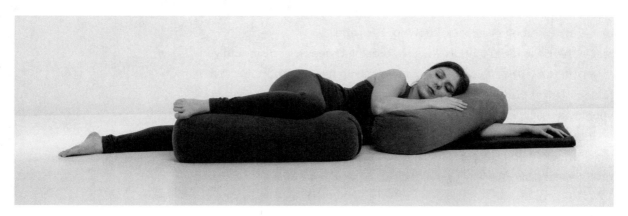

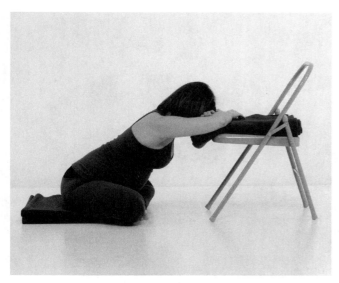

Sukhasana (Easy Seated Pose)

If you have time for only one pose, try this. Sit in Sukhasana (Easy Seated Pose) in front of a chair covered with a folded blanket. Extend through your spine and slowly lower your head to the chair seat. Using full, smooth breaths, bring your awareness to your belly. Stay in this pose as long as comfortable.

BENEFITS: Forward extensions with your head on a support cool your body and calm your nerves and allow your breath to flow more freely between your belly and throat.

MELISSA'S SEQUENCE FOR HIP AND PELVIC PAIN

MELISSA WILLIAMS

Depending on how your pain presents itself, some or all of these poses may offer you a degree of relief. Do not do any pose that causes you more pain or discomfort—hip or pelvic pain does not improve by overstretching.

Agni Stambhasana (Fire Log Pose)
Begin in Baddha Konasana (Bound Angle Pose). Slide the outer edge of your left shin onto the floor so your left heel is in front of your right hip. Pick up your right shin, allowing the weight to drop into your right knee, and place it on top of your left leg. Your right ankle should rest just beyond your left knee. Stay upright in the pose. Bring your hands in front of your shins and gently lift your heart forward, lengthening your spine and allowing your sitting bones to broaden. Breathe into your hips and gluteal muscles for several breaths. Slowly come out of the pose and reverse legs.

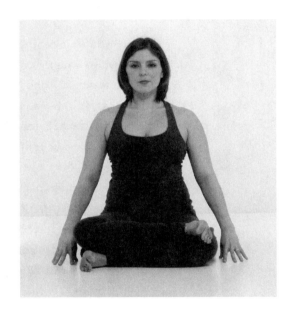

MODIFICATION: If your top knee is high in the air, don't stack your legs. Simply place your right shin in front of and parallel to the left.

BENEFIT: This action will create a nice stretch of the gluteal muscles without compressing your belly.

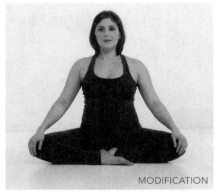

MODIFICATION

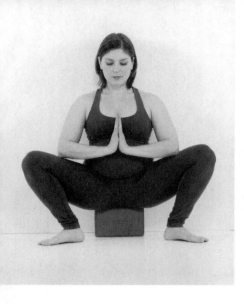

Malasana (Garland Pose)

Place a block against the wall. Come into a wide-legged squat with your body resting against the wall, your sitting bones on the block, and your hands in prayer position at your heart. Do not force your hips to rotate outward, and do not tuck your tailbone. Instead, gently allow each exhalation to help you soften through your pelvis and sacrum and through the gluteal muscles, which can pinch the sciatic nerve. Stay in this pose for one minute, if possible.

BENEFITS: This pose opens your hips and groin, releases your back muscles, and gently tones your abdominals without gripping.

Eka Pada Rajakapotasana (Pigeon Pose)

If you have time for only one pose, try this one. Start on your hands and knees or in Adho Mukha Svanasana (Downward-Facing Dog Pose). Move your right knee toward your right wrist and come into Eka Pada Rajakapotasana. Extend forward from your hips and release down toward the floor. Place your head on a block or a folded blanket for a more cooling experience. Remain in the pose for 5 to 10 breaths, or as long as comfortable. Slowly press back up and reverse legs.

MODIFICATIONS: If your right hip doesn't reach the mat, place a rolled blanket under it to bring balance to your sacrum. As your baby grows, you'll need to draw your front leg away from your body more to create a pocket for your belly, so you can extend your torso forward. Once your belly is pretty prominent, don't go all the way down; simply rest your head, chest, and forearms on a bolster placed in front of your bent leg.

BENEFITS: This pose releases tightness in your hips, deep gluteal muscles, groin, and psoas muscles, relieving impinged piriformis muscles and alleviating sciatica.

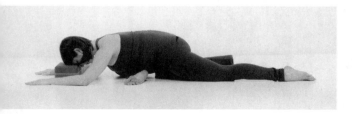

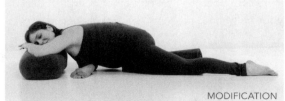

MODIFICATION

Nourishing Yourself

To have a healthy pregnancy—and birth a healthy baby—we need to make consciously healthy food choices. Yoga, of course, offers the best pregnancy "diet" by encouraging us to eat *sattvic* foods that are pure, easily digested, and filled with prana (life force) to nourish both mama and baby. In other words, you want a high-protein, mostly vegetarian diet with plenty of water to drink. A sattvic diet is similar to an anti-inflammatory diet, or what is known as the Mediterranean diet. It focuses on organic vegetables and fruits (the fresher the better); healthy fats (like avocados, olives, and nuts); whole grains without genetically modified organisms (GMOs); organic cow's milk or organic, unsweetened almond milk; and ample protein. If you maintain a vegetarian diet, eat plenty of quinoa, beans, legumes, and bulgur, as well as rice and dal. If you eat animal protein, stick to low-mercury fish (sardines, wild salmon, mackerel, anchovies) and high-quality cheese and yogurt, and eat organic chicken or grass-fed, grass-finished beef sparingly. Fresh foods imbued with prana and prepared with love bring vitality to your body and refresh your mind as well. Here's an easy way to remember what to have: eat fresh, real food, organic whenever possible; drink plenty of water; and stay away from any products laced with chemicals or artificial preservatives or with ingredients you can't pronounce.

It almost goes without saying, but cut out foods and beverages that you already know aren't healthy for your own body. According to ayurveda, alcohol, caffeine (in chocolate, energy drinks, and black teas as well as coffee), sugar, and super spicy foods are too stimulating for a mama-to-be and her baby. Processed, packaged, or canned foods have little nutritional value and additives that can be harmful, and many cans are still lined with bisphenol A (plastic).

If you do eat animal products, you'll want to approach your selections carefully. It's vital that you choose meat, eggs, and dairy from reputable sources to guard against ingesting antibiotics or pesticides. Buy organic, fresh, and unprocessed foods—with the exception of cheese, which should be pasteurized to guard against bacteria; steer clear of foods that have been genetically modified, like corn and soy; and don't buy prepackaged ground meats (grind your own). Fish should be low on the mercury scale (no tuna, shellfish, shark, or swordfish), and even sushi-grade raw fish should be avoided.

Some mamas feel better if they go gluten-, dairy-, and sugar-free. If you're one of them, substitute rice flour or flours made with amaranth, quinoa, or a mixture of gluten-free grains; use almond, soy, or rice milk; and try molasses instead of sugar.

Food Cravings

Pickles and ice cream for breakfast. Chocolate and popcorn with a side of bacon for an otherwise vegan mama. Mac and cheese at 3 A.M. Even if you've been uber-conscious of what you put in your mouth so far, food cravings are a real phenomenon, and some of them are pretty strange and insistent. Western researchers list several causes for these unusual desires. Some experts say we can blame our prenatal raging hormones for both the foods we crave and the foods that make us want to hurl, which are not that different from the foods we love and loath during PMS as well.

Others say we are drawn to what we need nutritionally (like fruits rich in vitamin C) and repelled by foods or beverages that might be harmful (like alcohol) or carry foodborne bacteria (like meat and seafood). Gina Sirchio, a chiropractor and certified clinical nutritionist in Chicago, says the body needs to load up on healthy fats to aid in the development of the baby's brain and central nervous system. She says sometimes pregnant women push aside the "healthy" part of that equation and turn to "ice cream and lots of cheese, and that's okay, too—in moderation." Jackie Keller, RD, a nutrition life coach and the author of *Body after Baby*, says it can actually be hard to distinguish between the body needing a specific nutrient and the mind simply craving something "because emotions run the gamut during pregnancy and often your psychological 'wants' escalate to physical 'gotta haves.'" One study notes that women have a heightened sense of bitter tastes in the first two trimesters, leading scientists to speculate that this awareness is "an evolutionary protection" that keeps us from inadvertently eating or drinking anything toxic.

Food cravings have been around as long as women have been conceiving and the ancient ayurvedic texts have an unusual, rather poetic explanation for such desires. They say that around the fourth month or so, the mother develops a "second heart" through which she receives needs and desires directly from her baby's heart. These communiqués from the baby to the *dauhrudini* (the "one with the two hearts") manifest as the mother's cravings. The ancients say women should always listen to those messages and give in to the cravings, because that will ensure the birth of a healthy baby. The classics go on to say that if wholesome foods and experiences do not satisfy the mother's cravings and the baby's desires, then it's fine to give in to the not-so-healthy ones—in moderation, of course.

Whose Body Is This? Staying Connected with Your Changing Body

Like most women, I couldn't wait to move from the first trimester into the second. I could string coherent thoughts together again almost seamlessly. I got to ditch the saltines in favor of fruits and oatmeal and sometimes even eggs in the morning. I stayed awake on the bus ride home after work. And yes, my hair looked great and my skin no longer had the greenish pallor of a sailor on her maiden voyage.

But something else happened, something I didn't expect. I hated how I looked: frumpy and misshapen. I remember going to a friend's out-of-town wedding when I was about five months along. I could still fit into my pre-pregnancy clothes—which were just a little more snug—so I only took regular clothes to wear. At the end of the long day-into-evening affair, I went back to the hotel. My dress strained to stay buttoned at the waistline, and my feet pressed against the constraints of my shoes. I couldn't get undressed fast enough. But when I looked at my naked body in the mirror, I didn't recognize the woman staring back at me. She didn't look pregnant; she looked—fat. I burst into tears. Where was my cute "bump"? What was going on in this trusted body of mine?

Looking back, I wish someone had told me that my distress was common. Apparently a lot of women have a hard time wrapping their heads around the need to gain weight while still living in a society that seems to beat us up for every pound we put on. A lifetime of being immersed in these not-so-subtle messages can do a number on women's self-esteem, especially if they have contended with full-blown eating disorders. From my "small picture" perspective, I had looked the same since I was about eighteen years old and didn't know how to relate to the rounder, softer woman I was quickly becoming. Looking at the big picture, of course, I knew in my heart that not only was this body change temporary, it was exactly what had to happen so I could birth a beautiful being into the world. My body had become someone else's home, and I needed to get over my hang-ups, and make that home the warmest, healthiest, most loving place possible. But that knowledge didn't make it any easier for me to adjust.

Pregorexia

Women who have suffered from anorexia or bulimia before they get pregnant are susceptible to a disorder called pregorexia. This fear of gaining weight often manifests in a woman restricting calories or exercising obsessively while pregnant. Taken to extremes, pregorexia can cause serious problems like intrauterine growth retardation or other neurological difficulties from lack of nutrients. While yoga has helped some women break free of this suffering, if you struggle with pregorexia, it's best to consult a therapist who is well versed in eating disorders and can help you shift your focus from your needs to your baby's. Also, be sure to let your midwife and doctor know about the problem so they can offer resources to help you.

A Body in Training

Those with any kind of body image challenges often find pregnancy difficult. One common reason women succumb to eating disorders (besides the obvious cultural fixation on excessively thin models and celebrities) is to gain a sense of control over one aspect of their lives when everything else happening around them seems to be out of their power. So they monitor what goes into their mouths, how many calories they burn, and how much weight they gain (or lose). They become obsessed with how they look. There's nothing like pregnancy to remind a woman that she really doesn't have control of everything—and that's okay, because she'll need to remember that when she becomes a mom.

Having a consistent yoga practice *before* you get pregnant will help you see the folly of your controlling ways. Erica Rodefer Winters, a writer and yoga teacher from Charleston, South Carolina, agrees. She learned that no matter how many green smoothies she drank, no matter how many times she visited BabyCenter.com, and no matter how much yoga she did or how often she meditated, she had no control over the actual process of growing her baby. "You just have to trust that your body knows what to do," she says. "I think learning to trust my body's cues during asana practice [before I got pregnant] really helped me to be okay with that."

I began to think of my pregnancy and all its tribulations and exaltations as a trial run of what my life might be like in nine months. A prolonged dress rehearsal for my baby and me. I knew I couldn't control how my baby would enter the world, no matter how much I planned and visualized ahead of time. And once she was born, how much control would I have over her sleeping, eating, and waking times anyway? Or my own, for that matter?

Yoga helps women—me included—switch our mind-set from the external to the internal, taking our focus off physical minutia and placing it on the collective whole. For example, we feel the steadiness of our arms in Downward-Facing Dog, the determination of our legs as we press our thighs up and back, the power of our breath to guide us within and between each pose. We connect with our strength and not our perceived flaws. And that strength, along with the ability to let go, will serve us well in the months ahead.

Yoga and meditation teacher Janice Gates says that when she got tangled up in negativity, she would turn to the Yoga Sutra, which encourages us to cultivate the opposite attitude. Instead of getting stuck on a destructive spinning wheel of thoughts (*What's wrong with my body? Why am I so grumpy? What's happened to me?*), see if you can flip those thoughts on their heads: *My body is a beautiful receptacle for creating and nurturing life. I am happy, I am healthy, and I am ready to embrace these life-giving changes*. Welcome your experience; honor your ability to create life; and go into the unknown with curiosity, patience, and devotion.

Several things helped me get over my body obsession. First, my belly finally popped out in front, which thrilled and relieved me—a visible and loving reminder that I was really pregnant, and the reason for all this added weight. Second, I felt my baby move, an experience that defies description. Third, I decided to dedicate my yoga practice to my baby. My internal inquiry became *How can I love my baby more?* and I consciously set an intention every morning to surrender to the experience of pregnancy—whatever showed up that day or even that moment. Fourth, I made a commitment to celebrate our time together in whatever small ways I could and to silence the annoying voices in my head that threatened to derail my joy. Finally, when I learned what my body was capable of doing physiologically to make all this happen, I was in awe.

Body Awareness Meditation

Sit in your favorite meditation position, using any props you need to be comfortable. With your eyes closed, bring your awareness to your face, softening your temples, forehead, cheekbones, and jaw. Move down to your throat, allowing your exhalations to release tension in your neck, the back of your neck, and your upper back and shoulders.

Now bring your awareness to your breasts, acknowledging with gratitude that they're growing to provide nourishment to your baby. Placing your hands on your belly, honor and welcome its ability to expand to provide a warm, safe place for your baby to grow. Shift your attention to your upper thighs, legs, and feet, celebrating their strength and their ability to hold you up. Sit quietly for another 5 to 10 minutes and give thanks to your whole body for being exactly the right size and shape to bring your baby into this world.

ROOTING DOWN AND LOOKING WITHIN: YOUR SECOND TRIMESTER PRACTICE

STEPHANIE SNYDER

Your practice through the rest of your pregnancy is about listening and discovering: What do you need right now? More energy or more rest? To create more space or to fold inward? As you transition from pose to pose, your breath will carry you through the easy, the awkward, and the challenging. Take time throughout this trimester to acquaint yourself with this very primitive, sacred, and courageous breath, which will serve you well during the birthing experience. Practice slow and conscious breathing until you are able to let your breath breathe you. Do as much or as little as you want, linking poses together or practicing them one by one.

Connection

Sit on a folded blanket or bolster so the top of your pelvis rocks slightly forward and your thighs release down; be sure you feel comfortable and relaxed and there is plenty of room for your belly. Allowing your outer pelvis to descend, lengthen your inner spine; without losing that length, soften and widen the back of your body. Place one hand on your heart and the other on your belly. Begin to breathe deeply and easily. Sense how your baby is sharing this quiet and peaceful moment with you now. The Upanishads describe the real self as a light that shines undisturbed within the windless cave of the heart. Gaze at that inner light now and recognize that you are full of life and full of light—yours and your baby's.

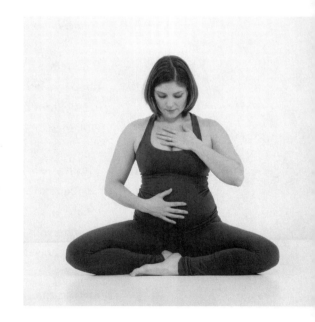

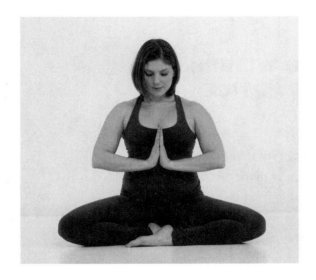

Intention

Bring your hands together in front of your heart and bow your head slightly toward your fingertips. The intention for this practice is to acknowledge yourself and your pregnancy with gratitude, to see yourself as an expression of grace, and to offer yourself a generous and loving embrace at this beautiful and intense time in your life. If the following intention resonates with you, allow it to set the tone and intention for your practice today:

This practice is a declaration of my gratitude. I recognize my ever-growing beauty and strength. I joyfully let go of any urge to judge myself or my efforts in any way. Today I will see the world the way I would like my baby to see it. I will see the goodness, the generosity, and the loving support that this life has to offer. May this practice be of great benefit to me, to my baby, and to all beings everywhere.

Return one hand to your heart and the other to your belly. Take a long, deep inhalation; as you exhale, sing the word OM. Let the sound fall like a lullaby from the universe to you and from you to your baby. You may chant OM once or several times.

Meditation/Pranayama

Continue sitting for 5 to 10 slow, deep breaths, feeling your upper lungs inflate as you inhale and the backs of your lungs release as you exhale. Breathe with your baby. Let the rhythm and length of your breath feel natural and nourishing now and throughout your practice.

Sukhasana (Easy Seated Pose) Variations

Sit with your sitting bones on the edge of a firm blanket with one shin in front of the other, and place your hands on your knees. Begin by arching your back and gently gazing up as you inhale, then rounding your back

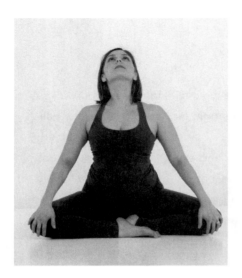 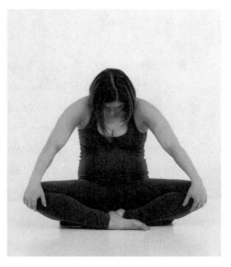

and gazing toward your baby as you exhale. Feel for the fullness in your upper chest on the inhalation and the fullness in your lower back on the exhalation, all the while gently rocking your baby forward and back. Do this as often as you like, then return to a neutral spine.

Begin to draw small circles with your spine. As you move from right to back to left to front, feel your sitting bones accommodate the motion by rocking very slightly in the same direction as your movements. Once you get the hang of it, make larger circles. Move 3 to 5 times in one direction; reverse your legs and draw circles in the other direction 3 to 5 times. Let the movement feel easy and fluid.

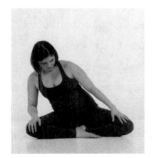 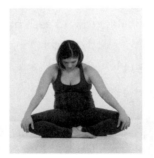 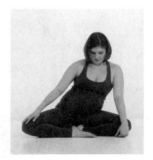 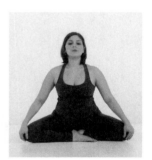

BENEFITS: These variations of Sukhasana release your spine and pelvic floor muscles, move your breath deep into your uterus, and provide a gentle rocking motion for your baby.

Calf Stretch

Come onto your hands and knees, with your shoulders over your wrists and your hips over your knees. Extend your right leg, back pressing the ball of your foot into the floor to open the calf muscles and back of that leg. After 3 breaths here, lift your right leg, and extend your left arm in front of you to no more than the torso height. Gently hugging your belly toward your spine, rotate your left wrist and right ankle 5 times in each direction to increase circulation in the joints. Return your knee and hand to the floor, and repeat on the other side.

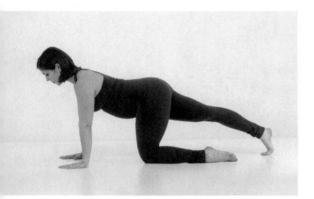 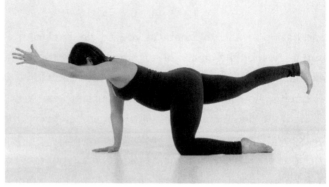

Tail Wag

Come back to your hands and knees and begin to wag your tail. Exhale your right hip and right shoulder toward each other as you gaze to the right; feel the left side of your body stretch. Inhale back to the center and exhale to the left. Complete this back-and-forth cycle several times

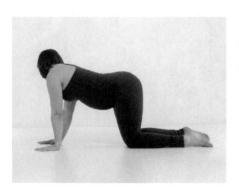 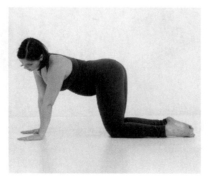 slowly. Finish by circling your pelvis several times in one direction and several times in the other, including your whole spine in the movement if it feels good. Move consciously but with freedom.

Uttana Shishosana (Extended Puppy Pose)

From your hands and knees, walk your hands forward, stretching your arms and lengthening the sides of your body as you drop your forehead to the floor. Keep your knees at least as wide as your hips. This is a good time to send your intention out into the universe. As you press your upper arms toward the floor, resist the action by moving your front ribs up into your body so the opening of your shoulders is integrated and there is no compression in your lower back. Remain in this pose for 5 breaths or more and then press back into Adho Mukha Svanasana (Downward-Facing Dog Pose).

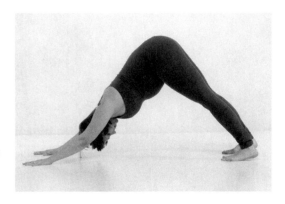

NOTE: This shoulder-opening, back-releasing pose can stand in as a substitute for Adho Mukha Svanasana anytime, especially on days when your energy flags.

**Adho Mukha Svanasana
(Downward-Facing Dog Pose)**

Your hands should be approximately shoulder-width apart and turned slightly outward so your shoulders can freely move away from your ears. Point your middle fingers toward the front corners of your mat to relieve any compression in your inner wrists, and place your feet slightly wider apart than your hips. Stay in this pose for several breaths, coming down into Balasana (Child's Pose) or Uttana Shishosana (Extended Puppy Pose) whenever you wish.

BENEFITS: This pose stretches your whole spine, releases tension in your neck and lower back, and lifts your baby off your pelvic floor. It can also be helpful in encouraging your baby to move into the optimal birthing position.

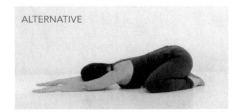

ALTERNATIVE

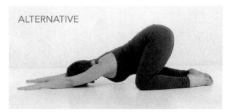

ALTERNATIVE

Moving through Vinyasa (optional)

If you're feeling energized, move from Adho Mukha Svanasana (Downward-Facing Dog Pose) to Phalakasana (Plank Pose) and back again 3 to 5 times and then lower down through Chaturanga Dandasana (Four-Legged Staff Pose) coming down to your knees, if you wish. Push up into Urdhva Mukha Svanasana (Upward-Facing Dog Pose) and then return to Adho Mukha Svanasana. Step forward into Uttanasana (Standing Forward Bend).

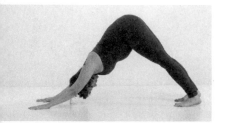
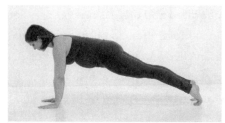
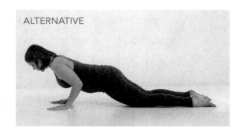

ALTERNATIVE

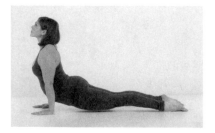
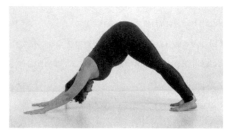

MODIFICATION: Use a bolster under your thighs as you move from Chaturanga Dandasana into Urdhva Mukha Svanasana to give your belly more room. If you feel any pressure or tightness in your belly, come to your hands and knees for Cat/Cow pose instead.

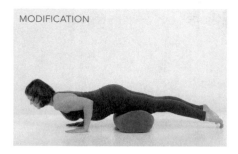

MODIFICATION

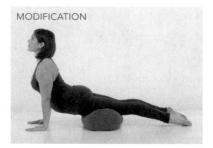

MODIFICATION

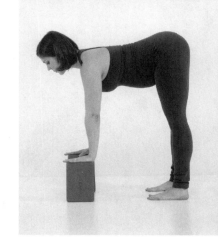

Uttanasana (Standing Forward Bend)

With your legs hip-width or more apart (depending on how large your belly is), lengthen your spine, keep your collarbones wide, and extend up through the sides of your body. Keeping your legs straight and strong, lift your inner groin back while directing your sitting bones toward your heels, and extending your spine forward. Place your hands on blocks placed far enough in front of your feet to leave plenty of room for your belly.

Virabhadrasana II (Warrior II Pose)

From Uttanasana (Standing Forward Bend), exhale your left foot back and open into Virabhadrasana II, extending your arms out to the sides. Inhale as you straighten your right leg and bring your hands into prayer position at your heart and exhale as you return to Virabhadrasana II. Repeat this flow of bending and straightening your front leg 3 times, then hold Virabhadrasana II for 3 to 5 more breaths with your arms in Garudasana (Eagle Pose). Return to Tadasana (Mountain Pose), then reverse legs and repeat the flow.

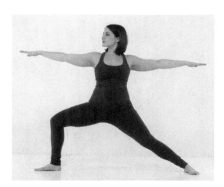
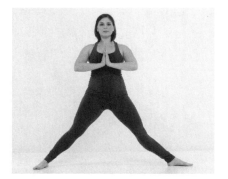
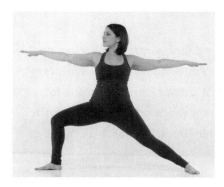
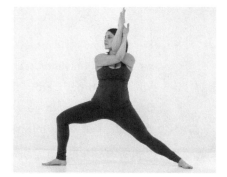

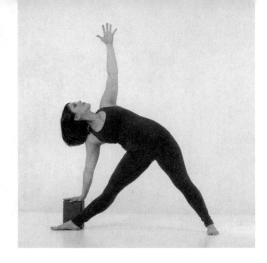

Utthita Trikonasana (Extended Triangle Pose)

From Tadasana (Mountain Pose), step your left foot back and come into Utthita Trikonasana, keeping both legs straight and strong. Use a block to create more space in the right side of your body so you don't compress the side of your belly or your lower back. Remain here for 3 to 5 slow, smooth, deep breaths. Repeat on the other side. Come back into Tadasana at the top of your mat.

Virabhadrasana II to Parsvakonasana (Warrior II Pose to Extended Side-Angle Pose) Vinyasa

Exhale your left foot back into Virabhadrasana II. Take a deep breath in and exhale into Viparita Virabhadrasana (Reverse Warrior Pose). Inhale back to center and exhale into Utthita Parsvakonasana, placing your right elbow on your right thigh (or your hand on a block) and your left arm over your head.

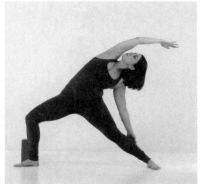
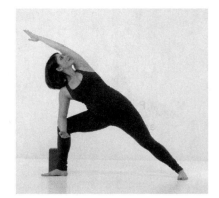

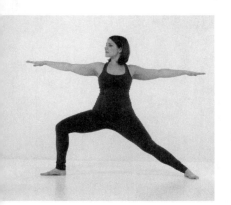

Do this flow—Virabhadrasana II to Viparita Virabhadrasana to Utthita Parsvakonasana and back again—3 times, moving with your breath. Hold the last Utthita Parsvakonasana for 3 to 5 breaths with your left arm wrapped around your body to grab your right thigh in a half-bind. Repeat this vinyasa on the other side.

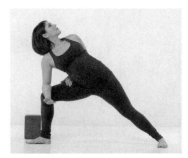

Utkata Konasana (Goddess Pose) Vinyasa

Starting in a wide stance, with your feet as wide apart as is comfortable, bend your knees and hold Utkata Konasana for 3 breaths. Inhale as you straighten your legs, reaching your arms over your head. As you exhale, bend your knees and bring your arms down, bending them at the elbows into a cactus shape. Do this flow 5 times. On the last round, commit to the final Utkata Konasana for 3 breaths.

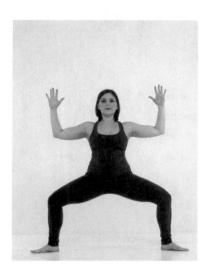 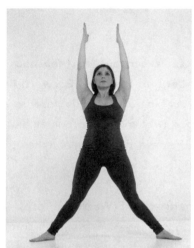 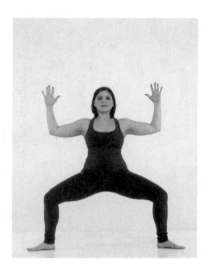

Prasarita Padottanasana (Wide-Legged Standing Forward Bend)

From Utkata Konasana (Goddess Pose), straighten your legs and move your feet so they are parallel to each other. Extend your torso forward, placing your hands on blocks. Keeping your buttocks over your legs, lengthen your upper body—as in Adho Mukha Svanasana (Downward-Facing Dog Pose)—to release your spine and open your shoulders and hamstrings. Stay in this pose for several breaths, or as long as it feels comfortable.

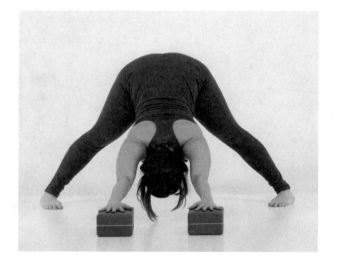

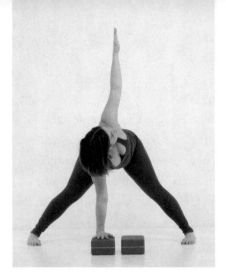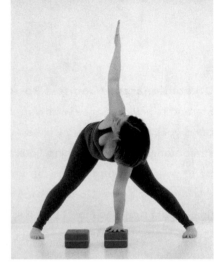

Parivrtta Prasarita Padottanasana (Wide-Legged Standing Forward Bend) with Twist

Bring your blocks and hands closer to your feet. With your right hand on the block, twist and reach your left arm up toward the sky for a breath or two. Release, then repeat on the other side. Return to center before coming up to standing.

Virabhadrasana I (Warrior I Pose)

Standing with legs in Prasarita Padottanasana (Wide-Legged Standing Forward Bend), turn your right foot out and your left foot in; come into Virabhadrasana I. Exhale your arms behind your back, either holding on to your elbows or coming into reverse prayer position. Hold the pose for 3 to 5 breaths, release, and repeat on the other side.

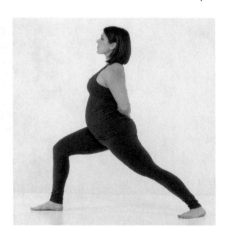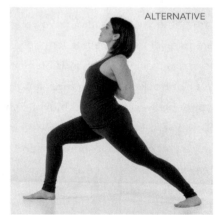

ALTERNATIVE

Uttanasana (Standing Forward Bend)

From Virabhadrasana I (Warrior I Pose), step your back foot up to meet your front foot at the top of your mat. Extend forward into a long, lifted Uttanasana, with your hands on blocks placed far enough in front of you to lengthen your torso. Stay here for 3 to 5 breaths before coming down to your hands and knees.

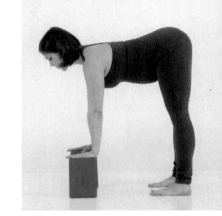

One-Legged Hip Circles

Starting on your hands and knees, bring your right foot forward to the outside of your right hand. With your knees bent at 90 degrees and your hands under your shoulders, begin to create big circles with your entire pelvis. This is a big rocking motion. If you would like to, you can place your forearms on the floor to ease any lower back tension as well. Do hip circles 5 to 7 times and then reverse legs and repeat on the other side. Move into Adho Mukha Svanasana (Downward-Facing Dog Pose) for a few breaths.

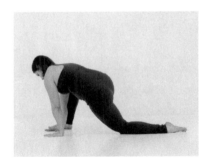
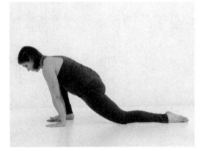
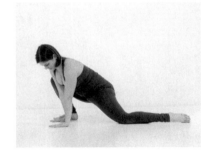

ALTERNATIVE

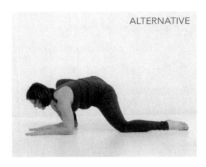
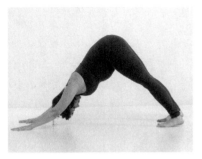

BENEFITS: This pose can help open your pelvis to make room for the baby to descend and release any tension in your hips.

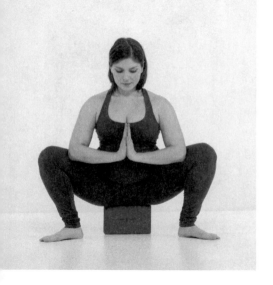

Malasana (Garland Pose)

From Adho Mukha Svanasana (Downward-Facing Dog Pose), begin to walk your hands back toward your feet. Have your block nearby. Bend your knees to come into a wide-kneed squat, placing the block at medium height directly under your sitting bones. If you feel unstable, do this pose against the wall. Your feet should be flat on the floor and turned outward slightly, and your knees should point in the same direction as your feet. Allow your pelvis to descend onto the block as you lift and lengthen your spine. Bring your hands together in prayer position at your heart, and take several deep, soothing breaths.

BENEFITS: This pose can help position the baby in your pelvis and open your hips as your baby grows.

NOTE: Acknowledge that you can be both strong and supple at the same time—the *sthira* and *sukha* of motherhood. You may very well give birth in this position a few months from now, so take time to do some positive affirmation and visualization while you are here.

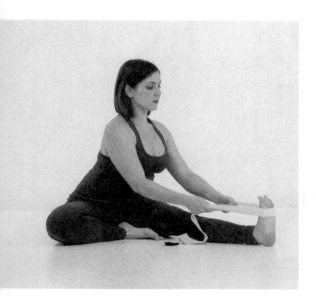

Janu Sirsasana (Head-on-Knee Pose)

Sit up on a blanket if necessary so you can maintain the natural curve in your lower back. Straighten your left leg out in front of you and place the sole of your right foot against your left inner thigh. Pause here and let the tops of your femurs become heavy and rooted. Then lift your spine, sending your sternum toward the sky. Loop a strap around your left foot, and hold onto the strap with both hands. Pulling back on the strap, begin to move your chest forward without compressing your belly at all. Engage your left quadricep muscles enough to feel a stretch in your hamstrings but not so much as to lift your heel or lock your knee. Keep your collarbones wide and the whole pose energized. Stay here for 5 breaths. Reverse legs and repeat.

BENEFITS: This pose strengthens your spine and legs and tones your uterus.

Sukhasana (Easy Seated Pose) Twist

Sit in a modified Sukhasana with your sitting bones elevated on a folded blanket. Instead of crossing your legs at the ankles—which could contribute to swelling toward the end of your second trimester—place your right calf directly in front of your left shin. Square your hips and begin twisting to your right. Bring your right hand to the floor behind you and place your left hand on your right knee or in front of your shin. Keep the twist in your upper spine, chest, and back; stay here for 3 breaths. Reverse legs and repeat the twist to the left side.

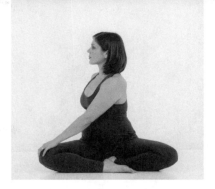

CAUTION: If you feel a pulling sensation along your lower back or belly, ease out of the pose.

BENEFITS: This pose opens your upper back, broadens your chest, and releases your neck and shoulders.

MODIFICATION

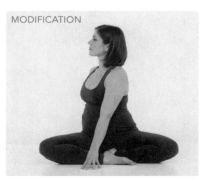

Baddha Konasana (Bound Angle Pose)

Sitting with the soles of your feet together and your knees apart, bring your hands behind you and lift your belly and heart to create as much space between your belly and pelvic floor as possible. Begin to walk your hands forward, keeping your arms straight like kickstands. Come forward only a few inches, leaving plenty of space for your baby. Instead of folding forward, extend your spine, keeping the front of your spine long and your heart open. Stay here for several breaths or as long as you're comfortable.

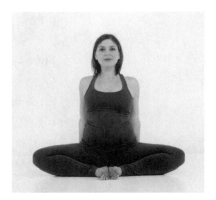

MODIFICATION: If you are less flexible, stay upright with your hands behind you, and let the opening of your chest bring in a bigger breath as your thighs drop down.

BENEFITS: This pose broadens your pelvis, strengthens your spine, and improves your posture. In Baddha Konasana, you can also release and lift your pelvic floor muscles and gently tone your abdominals without gripping.

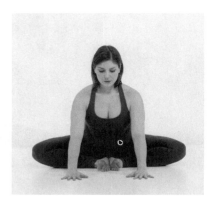

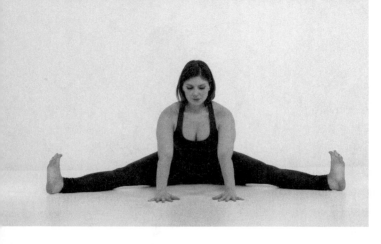

Upavistha Konasana (Wide-Angle Seated Pose)

Sit with your legs straight out in front of you and spread them only wide enough to feel a stretch in your hamstrings but not in your inner knees. If you do feel your inner knees, bring your legs closer together. Walk your hands forward until you feel a lengthening in your spine without compressing your belly. Engage your legs with your toes pointing straight up. With your arms in front of you, push the floor away to rock your weight back onto your sitting bones. This creates balance and stability within the stretch. Stay here for 5 breaths, then slowly come out.

CAUTION: If you feel any pressure in your pelvis or any pain at all, pull your legs closer together or omit the pose.

BENEFITS: This pose improves the circulation in your legs, releases your pelvic floor muscles, and energizes your whole body.

Side-Lying Savasana (Modified)

Lying on your left side, straighten your left leg. Bend your right leg and place the knee, shin, and foot on a bolster that you've positioned in front of and parallel to your straight left leg. (Don't put the bolster between your legs; only under the top, bent knee.) Rest your head on a bolster or folded blanket so that it's in line with your spine. Remain in the pose for as long as you like, at least 3 to 5 minutes.

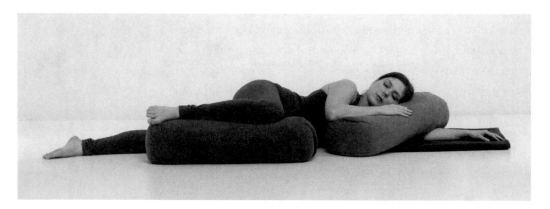

BENEFITS: This restorative pose soothes your nervous system and gives you deep rest, which can restore your energy and quell any signs of anxiety.

Meditation

Come to a comfortable seated position, close your eyes, and place your hands on your belly. Allow your breath to move your attention inward. Placing your attention on your baby, spend 5 to 10 minutes (or as long as you like) breathing gratitude and love to your little one (and to yourself).

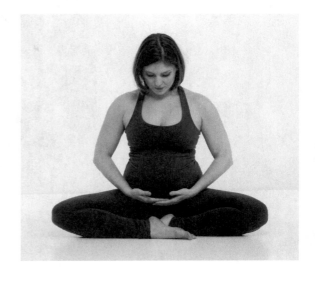

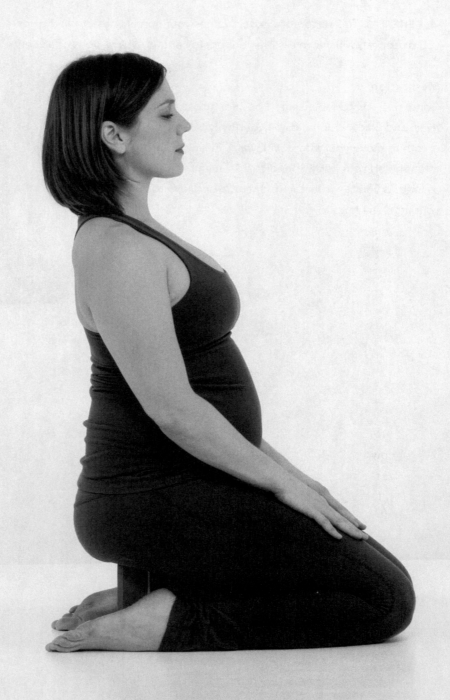

3.

THE PELVIC FLOOR

*Toning, Releasing, and Preparing
for Labor throughout Your Pregnancy*

Sequences by Jane Austin

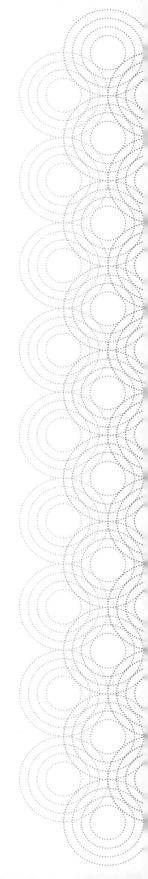

As yoga practitioners, we spend a good part of our lives actively *in* our bodies. We use the breath to move us from pose to pose. We lift up through the pelvic floor by gently engaging the *bandhas*—the seals or locks that keep our focus and energy in the body. And we pride ourselves in knowing what our bodies are capable of and what their limitations are. So logic would dictate that giving birth should be relatively easy for us.

Unfortunately that's not the case for a lot of yoginis. I never would have believed it, but several years ago, I had a conversation with Donna, a well-known yoga teacher from Oakland, California, that changed my mind. She told me she labored for fifty hours before giving birth to her first baby. How could that be? She did yoga—a lot. And yoga is a body-based practice that helps us get to know our bodies more intimately. While Donna credits her practice for her ability to withstand the prolonged pain, it was still fifty hours! So what happened? Donna told me she simply did not know how to release her pelvic floor. Her body didn't seem to know what that meant. And her experience is far from unique.

Something similar happened to Stephanie, who contributed sequences in Chapter 2: she endured twenty-two hours of hard labor during the birth of her first child. Margi, a yoga teacher based in San Francisco and New York City, struggled for thirty-six hours. What's going on here? Apparently all that lifting up and engaging the pelvic floor muscles gives many yoga practitioners not only buns of steel but pelvic floors of iron. Overly aggressive Mula Bandhas (Root Locks) and determined Kegel exercises—as well as anxiety and poor on- and off-the-mat posture—created hypertonic (overly tight) pelvic floors. Not to mention that all the stories out there of postpartum incontinence and permanently prolapsed organs could be enough to scare any pregnant woman into doing the "tighten up," regardless of the real condition of her pelvic organs.

Far too many birth educators, pregnancy websites, and prenatal yoga teachers still encourage Kegels (or "diamonds and rubies" as the pelvic floor educator Leslie Howard calls them) several times a day. During Margi's pregnancy, everyone—even her shiatsu therapist—championed the benefits of Kegels. So Margi did "hundreds of diamonds and rubies, with effort and fervor, every single day. I drew the diamond of muscles that makes up the pelvic floor in and up and in and up and . . . in and up." She was so successful at strengthening and tightening her pelvic floor that her cervix opened only three centimeters in thirty-six hours. Her midwife, who had delivered close to two thousand babies in her career, peered over her glasses at Margi and sighed, "Oh no, another yoga teacher with a tight pelvic floor." In other words, says Margi, "Garage door jammed closed, baby stuck inside, and C-section looming."

How is it that we yoginis can engage our pelvic floor but don't seem to know how to release it? Even yoga teachers who study Western anatomy along with yoga's subtle anatomy seem to have trouble. What part of "letting go" eludes us? I think it's a question of balance and connection. First of all, we sometimes overemphasize the upward movement of the in-breath (*prana vayu*) at the expense of the downward movement of the out-breath (*apana vayu*) and muscular contractions over muscular release. We do the same thing when we become obsessed with Kegeling. Second, far too many yoga teachers and students tuck their pelvises in a pose, which keeps the muscles in a constant state of tension and makes releasing them nearly impossible. Third, we're not always as conscious of the connection between the pelvic floor and the rest of the body as we could be. In fact, Jane Austin, the San Francisco–based prenatal teacher who provided expert advice in this chapter, says she's pretty surprised by how little her students know about their "lady parts." She has reason to be worried, because this disconnect can have a profound, lifelong impact on our health and well-being. It may explain why so many women like Donna and Stephanie have prolonged labors during their first pregnancies and much quicker results in subsequent births. Stephanie says her second birthing experience was easier not only because "the gates had been softened and opened during the previous" birth, but also "the bumpy road of uncertainty had been paved with insight."

Smoothing that bumpy road means connecting with your pelvic floor, but that's difficult to do when so many women have no idea "what's up down there." Like Margi, we're told to do Kegels and more Kegels without any explanation of how those muscles relate to the rest of the pelvic floor or to the body as a whole. The ability to tone and release the pelvic floor is so vital to a healthy pregnancy and a natural, joyous birthing experience that I chose to give it its own chapter and share it with you well before labor begins.

Kegels and Other Exercises

Kegels should not take all the blame for women's locked-up pelvises. Arnold Kegel, MD, never designed his eponymous pelvic floor exercises as a one-way street; in fact, he instructed his patients to release their pelvic floor muscles as often as they squeeze them. The contraction should be a gentle lift—not a vice grip. Also, exercises for the pelvic floor should engage more than just the urethra muscles. So the cue many doctors give their patients—stopping and then restarting the flow of urine—is incorrect. We also need to contract and then release the muscles in the center of the pelvis around the vagina and the anus.

Just hearing the directive "Do your Kegels" conjures up a rather determined way of finding and engaging your pelvic floor, so Jane Austin prefers to separate pelvic floor exercises from the name Kegel. But she does agree that these exercises can benefit women, especially those who have "low-tone pelvic muscles" (hypotonia) and stress incontinence.

Even if you have a high-toned (hypertonic) pelvic floor, you can still benefit from Kegels, but *only if you can feel the release of the muscles after you engage them*. Most yoga practitioners (and dancers and Pilates instructors as well) experience tightness not just in the superficial muscles but in the deeper ones—the levator ani in particular—that help protect and support the pelvic organs (the bladder, uterus, vagina, and rectum). "Contracting an already contracted muscle," Jane says, "can make releasing and opening the pelvic floor much more difficult." And ironically, it only makes the muscle weaker, not stronger.

Women need flexible strength in the pelvis—not too tight, not too loose. Just like in yoga, pelvic floor muscles must be able to soften and stretch around the baby as he moves through the birth canal. When the muscles are too tight and weak, they don't stretch very well and can cause trauma to the muscle tissue—and a great deal of pain for the mother. Low-tone muscles, on the other hand, may be too loose to support the baby as he moves into the correct position for birth and could even cause the pelvic organs to prolapse.

When you tuck your tailbone in yoga poses (or as a postural choice in everyday life), your pelvic floor muscles scoop, lift, and grip along with your gluteal (butt) muscles. By forcing your sacrum toward the front of your body, this tucking action increases tension in your pelvis, as well as in your hips and glutes. So don't tuck your tailbone and don't suck in your belly—good advice for nonpregnant women too. Instead, practice muscle-lengthening exercises to stretch your calves, hamstrings, psoas muscles, and adductors (inner thigh muscles) to reestablish your lumbar curve, and learn how to hold your pelvis correctly.

Katie Bowman, a biomechanical scientist who founded the Restorative Exercise Institute in San Diego, has a valuable lesson for maintaining proper pelvic floor placement anytime: "Point your urethra toward the floor. Think about it. You don't pee out in front of you, do you? You pee straight down." Now when I think about my pelvic floor, I ask myself two questions: *Would I be able to pee properly in this position?* and *Do I still have a lumbar curve?*

More Than Muscle: A Part of a Whole

Sometimes our inability to let go doesn't necessarily signal hypertonia as much as it suggests a disconnect between our brain and our pelvis. No matter what condition your pelvic muscles are in, simply focusing on contracting or releasing an isolated set of muscles won't really do you much good. You need get the bones and tissue in your pelvis involved as well as the surrounding muscles. The whole system—muscles, bones, and tissue—must work together in a concerted way. In his book *Pelvic Power*, the pelvic floor expert Eric Franklin explains that this "interplay of the parts of the whole structure, not isolated muscle power, is what is crucial" for effective and flexible strength. And strength is never synonymous with tension. A chronically tense muscle is an exhausted and ultimately weakened one. It's like walking around all day flexing your bicep. When you finally release it, it feels tired and sore. If you were to engage it again, you might notice that it felt weaker. When the pelvic floor muscles are weak (causing stress incontinence when laughing, coughing, or running), the body compensates by gripping the gluteal muscles and adductors to keep the bladder closed.

B.K.S. Iyengar has essentially said the same thing as Franklin through the language of yoga. When we focus exclusively on one part of the body, we cause it great harm—the opposite of *ahimsa* (nonharming), the golden rule of yoga. How? By overgripping, going beyond our capabilities, forcing our way into a pose, or requiring one side of the body (or one set of muscles) to bear the brunt of holding us up. But Iyengar has also said that we harm the parts of the body we *don't* focus on—by not moving the breath into those areas, not noticing how the pose is affecting them, and not feeling a sense of gratitude for their participation.

In essence, we may have done great harm to our pelvic floor muscles by forcing them into a hypertonic state. And we've damaged the other bones, muscles, joints, and ligaments that make up or surround the pelvis through misalignment and lack of awareness. Interestingly enough, both Iyengar and pelvic floor experts tell us that we send our pelvic floor muscles into grip mode not only when we consciously do Kegels or tuck the pelvis, but also when we tighten our jaw, eyes, throat, shoulders, and even our brain (the yogic way of saying we exert too much effort). Of course, the reverse is true as well. Any gripping in the pelvis causes tension in the brain, jaw, eyes, shoulders, and throat.

The problem, naturally, is that many women—even yoga practitioners—don't know what else is down there besides their Kegel muscles. By isolating those muscles and focusing solely on their function, we do our bodies a great disservice and set ourselves up for problems—both before and after giving birth—because as Eric Franklin explains, the pelvic floor supports almost every movement we make. How can we learn to let go of something we don't even know we're holding on to? To understand how these muscles, bones, and organs work together to allow for smooth childbirth, we need to get better acquainted with the pelvic floor.

An Anatomy Lesson

Taking some time to visualize your pelvis will help you understand its vital role in pregnancy, labor, and birthing and learn how a healthy pelvis can create a healthy birthing experience. Made up of four bones, this diamond-shaped structure contains an opening called the pelvic outlet, through which your baby will descend as she enters the world. The pubic bone in front, the coccyx (tailbone) in back, and the sitting bones on the sides form the cornerstones of the pelvic outlet. The ilia, the two big side bones, meet at the pubic bone in front and at the coccyx in back. Ligaments, most notably the symphysis pubis in front and those that support the sacroiliac joints in back, connect these four bones. Several muscles also get involved and allow the bones of the pelvis to move slightly: the coccygeus muscles, the levator ani muscle, the parietal layer, and the visceral layer all protect and support the pelvic organs and their sphincters as well as the intestines and keep things in place even when we cough, sneeze, or laugh too vigorously. Even before they get pregnant, many women find taking a weekly yin yoga class—being careful not to overstretch the ligaments—can help keep the connective tissue well lubricated, which allows the muscles to slide and move in healthy ways.

Although it doesn't seem like the pelvis moves, it does. If it didn't, we wouldn't be able to move our legs or spine. It doesn't move much (in women who aren't pregnant), but small, subtle movements can create big changes throughout the whole body. As Eric Franklin says, a small shift in the pelvis can mean a big twist in the neck, the spine, or even the feet. As B.K.S. Iyengar pointed out, the position of the feet and the jaw, in turn, can negatively or positively influence the pelvis.

If your pelvis didn't move, you wouldn't be able to give birth. In fact, the hormones relaxin and progesterone, along with fluid retention, cause the pelvis to become quite mobile during pregnancy, which strengthens the organs and tissues and ramps up their blood supply. You need to be mindful of how much you stretch your muscles because, while relaxin allows your pelvis to open more, making space for your baby to move down and out, it can also create very flexible and often unstable joints.

Finding a Balance

Put simply, a well-functioning pelvis holds stuff in and lets stuff out with just the right amount of lift and release—not too tight, not too loose. A too-loose pelvis invites stress incontinence and even pelvic organ prolapse, which is when one or more of the pelvic organs collapses into the vagina. While many factors—such as genetics, hormonal changes, and poor nutrition—conspire to create these conditions, damaged or weakened pelvic floor muscles also contribute. Although organ prolapse can occur in natural or even gentle childbirth, it is less likely to happen if the mother can direct her baby through the pelvis herself in tune with her own rhythm and without bearing down or holding her breath.

How can you tell if you have a problem with your pelvic floor muscles? Pelvic floor dysfunction can surface before pregnancy—or even many years later—as pain in the hips, lower back, coccyx, pubic bone, or sacroiliac joints, and it can make penetration during sex quite uncomfortable. Past physical and emotional trauma, abuse issues, and even prior pelvic organ prolapse can all contribute to a hypertonic pelvis.

How Yoga Helps

When we truly practice vinyasa yoga, it can support and encourage a natural childbirth experience and a less painful (and hopefully shorter) labor. The very definition of vinyasa—placing in a special way (*vi*, meaning "to place"; *nyasa*, meaning "special way")—encourages us to bring our attention, our breath, and the highest aspect of our consciousness (our intuitive mind) to bear on what we're doing. Returning to this definition helps remind us that vinyasa is more than "workout yoga"; it allows us to place our attention on our experience and move according to what we need at any given moment. Directing your awareness inward—even when you have a strong, physical practice— gives you the opportunity to notice and celebrate the connectedness of the muscles, bones, joints, and ligaments throughout your body. Grip your jaw or tense your shoulders. Can you feel a corresponding tension in your pelvic floor? When you release your pelvic floor, can you feel a softening in your upper body? When you do a wide-legged standing pose, is the stretch in your groin too intense or just right? Yoga not only helps you tune in physically, but it allows you to bring the power of your breath, mind, and intuitive nature to every moment. Engaging all of the *koshas* every time you practice will help you notice these connections and use them to open the channels of your body and release your mind of any lingering fears.

If you can, start working with your pelvic floor before you get pregnant or at least as soon as you can. You'll likely find it a lot easier to visualize and work with the muscles, bones, and ligaments before your baby is pressing his head against them with a sense of urgency. Think of the asanas and breathing techniques described in this chapter as a way of befriending your pelvic floor. Incorporating them into your daily routine will prepare you for labor and birthing and give your baby enough room to settle into the right position comfortably for a smooth transition out. Remember, if your muscles are too tense, the space your baby has to move into will be constricted, and your hopes of having a natural childbirth will be dashed. That's because he won't have enough room to engage his whole head in the opening and so won't be able to dilate the cervix enough to get his head, shoulders, and body through. Equally important, becoming more intimate with your pelvic floor will help you better understand how to knit things back together after you give birth.

Discovering Your Pelvis

To figure out how to release their pelvic floor muscles, Jane Austin has her students spend some time actually feeling the bony structure of the pelvic outlet. Here is how she suggests you can explore this area.

Stand with your feet about hip-width apart or slightly wider. With your toes pointed forward, bend your knees. Place one hand on the front of your pelvis at the pubic bone and one hand on the back of your sacrum with your middle finger reaching toward the tip of your coccyx. As you tilt your pelvis forward and stick your bottom out, feel your sacrum move away from your pubic bone, your sitting bones spread, and your pelvic outlet widen. Now tuck your pelvis by moving your coccyx toward your pubic bone. In this position, your lower back flattens out and your sitting bones draw slightly closer together. Tilt your pelvis forward and back a few times to see how the movement affects the space at the outlet.

Now stick your bum out, reach around, and grab your sitting bones. If they elude you, put one foot on a chair, bend that knee, and try again. Notice how the pelvic outlet is more spacious when your pelvis is in a forward tilt.

The Dos and Don'ts of Squatting

Every prenatal yoga teacher encourages her students to do squats, squats, and more squats. Why? Because squatting widens the sitting bones and lengthens the muscles in the pelvis, which gives the baby room to move into the right birthing position. Squatting particularly benefits women with hypertonic pelvic floor muscles, but only if it's done right. Follow these tips:

- *Do* maintain a neutral or slightly forward tilt to your pelvis when you squat.
- *Don't* round your back when squatting—that can make it difficult for your baby's head to enter the top of your pelvis.
- *Do* include one-sided squats in your practice (see pages 163–64 in Chapter 4)
- *Don't* do deep squats in your last few weeks of pregnancy if your baby is not yet engaged in the right position (head down, facing your back). See Chapter 4 for a more detailed discussion about this.

Instead of doing Kegels aggressively, engage and release your pelvic floor the yogic way: by using your breath to ensure that your movements are gentle and complete. In this technique, the lift of the pelvic floor muscles actually happens on the exhalation, while the inhalation encourages the muscles to release. This rather counterintuitive breathing makes sense when you consider that the diaphragm moves down on the inhalation and lifts on the exhalation. As you inhale, feel your pelvic floor muscles release toward the floor. As you exhale, lift these muscles up very gently, without engaging your abdominal muscles, as if to keep a feather lifted. As the muscles lift and tighten on the exhalation, the urethra, vaginal opening, and anus will close, and you should feel a little tightening right above your pubic bone. The muscles should then release down as you inhale. You must able to both engage and release your pelvic floor muscles.

Sitting on an exercise ball is another great way to assess your muscle tone in this area. Feel your sitting bones on the ball. As you inhale, release your pelvic floor muscles down onto the ball. As you exhale, gently lift the muscles away from the ball.

NOTE: If you don't feel your pelvic floor muscles move down and up as you inhale and exhale, you may find working with a pelvic floor physical therapist helpful.

The Second (or Third or Fourth) Time Around

Are subsequent births really easier—and by easier, I mean shorter? Often but not always, so don't feel bad if your second birthing experience is harder and longer. Here's what the experts say:

- Your abdominal and pelvic floor muscles may be overstretched and weaker the second time around, which means your labor may be quicker and a little more insistent.
- Your uterus may not have shrunk to its pre-baby size, so your next baby may start growing sooner—and chances are you will feel her move sooner too.
- You and your cervix know what to do, and your body doesn't instinctively resist as much as it may have the first time around. In fact, the cervical and vaginal tissues may yield more readily to the baby's head, helping you push her out more quickly and easier.
- You may have more of the silent but effective Braxton Hicks contractions in subsequent pregnancies, which will allow your cervix to dilate and spread more quickly, helping to shorten labor.

PRACTICES FOR GETTING ACQUAINTED WITH YOUR PELVIC FLOOR

JANE AUSTIN

Maintaining proper posture and breathing will help you be more comfortable and have fewer physical complaints throughout your pregnancy; it will also set you up for an easier birthing experience. Let's start with good posture.

Proper Posture

The correct sitting position activates the pelvic floor by engaging the deep abdominals. Conversely, a slumped, rounded posture sends the body's weight into the sacrum, which recruits the more superficial abdominals and puts pressure on the pelvic floor.

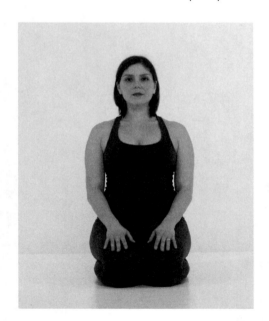

If you can maintain the natural curvature in your low back, sit on the floor in Virasana (Hero Pose). If you have tight hips and hamstrings that cause you to slump and round, sit at the edge of a chair instead, with your feet flat on the floor.

Maintain a connection between your sitting bones and the surface you are sitting on. To do this, first rock back and forth on your sitting bones and then move side to side. Begin to make small circles with your pelvis so that you feel the bones of your pelvis as well as the muscles between the bones.

Come to rest in the center of your sitting bones. From here, lengthen your spine and reach up through the crown of your head. Just sitting like this will improve most women's pelvic health.

Belly Breathing

Breathing into your belly will help you understand the connection between your pelvic floor and your diaphragm, which move together.

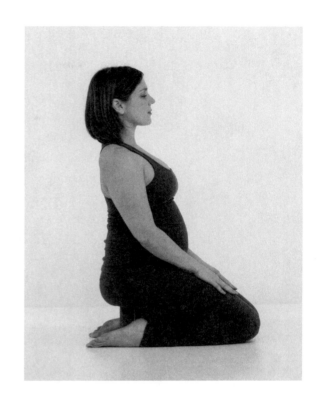

Remain in Virasana (Hero Pose), close your eyes, and begin breathing in and out through your nose. Now turn your attention to your pelvis. As you inhale, feel your thoracic diaphragm descend and your pelvic floor muscles release downward; as you exhale, notice that your diaphragm and pelvic floor come up. This very gentle movement should not create any gripping in your belly. Nor should it recruit your six-pack muscles (the rectus abdominus), which would create too much downward pressure on your pelvic floor muscles. As you breathe, allow your belly and lower ribs to expand and release, but keep your shoulders completely relaxed. If you have trouble feeling the diaphragm-pelvis connection, try exhaling through your mouth instead of your nose.

Be careful not to pull your belly in. This causes your shoulders to lift and inhibits the movement of the diaphragm. Do Belly Breathing for 10 to 15 minutes a day.

BENEFITS: Exploring the link between your pelvic floor and your breath helps you improve your ability to release your pelvic floor muscles during birth and tone those muscles after your baby arrives. Many women also find that Belly Breathing helps them sleep.

NOTE: To get the most benefit from Belly Breathing, begin this practice as soon as you discover you're pregnant; it gets trickier as the baby grows and restricts your diaphragm's ability to move.

Polar Bear Pose with Pelvic Tilts

Begin on your hands and knees. Lower your forearms to the floor, knees hip-width apart or slightly wider to make room for your baby. Press your forearms into the floor and release your head down. Visualize your baby resting in your belly hammock. As you breathe into your belly, stick your bum out, widen your sitting bones, and visualize your pelvic floor muscles lengthening. On an exhalation, tuck your pelvis and draw your coccyx toward your pubic bone; the muscles deep within your pelvis will contract slightly. Coordinate the movement and breath. As you inhale, visualize the muscle fiber of your pelvic floor lengthening and releasing, and as you exhale, tuck your pelvis and feel those muscles contracting. Rock your pelvis back and forth 8 to 10 times to the rhythm of your breath.

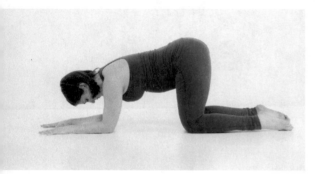 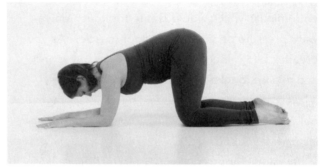

NOTE: Confine the movement to your pelvis and lower back, keeping your upper and middle back relatively still. When you're done, take a rest in Balasana (Child's Pose), with your knees wide, big toes together, and hips pressed back toward your feet.

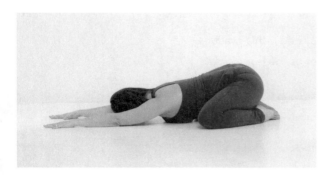

BENEFITS: Antigravity postures, such as Polar Bear Pose, can be effective tools for locating your pelvic floor muscles. This pose is especially helpful later in pregnancy as it can help relieve back pain and discomfort in your pelvis.

PELVIC TILTS, HIP CIRCLES, AND FIGURE EIGHTS

The poses in this three-part mini sequence can be done separately or flow together as a vinyasa sequence.

Pelvic Tilts

Come onto your hands and knees with your wrists under your shoulders and your knees under your hips (or slightly wider if your baby needs more room). Breathe normally, and begin to tip your pelvis forward and back. Confine the movement to your pelvic floor and find the depth of movement that feels good. With your inhalation, visualize your sitting bones spreading as your coccyx and pubic bones move apart. With each exhalation, tuck your pelvis and feel a gentle toning of your lower abdominal muscles.

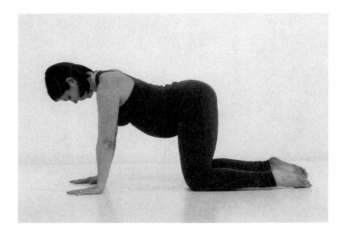 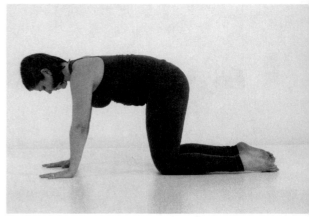

BENEFITS: This movement helps safely mobilize the joints that stabilize your sacrum.

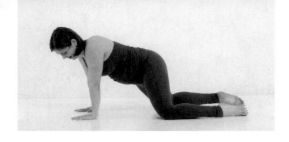

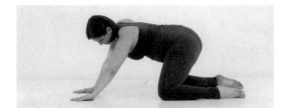

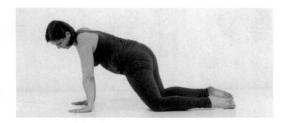

Hip Circles

Remain on your hands and knees. Close your eyes. As you visualize your baby resting comfortably in your belly, begin to make circles with your hips. Start small and gradually make the circles bigger. Now widen your knees a little, gently inhale your hips forward, and around to the right; exhale as you press your hips back toward your feet and around to the left. The movement should free any tension in your hips and back. Continue the circles several times in one direction and several times in the other.

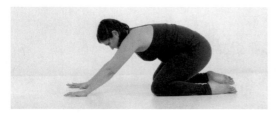

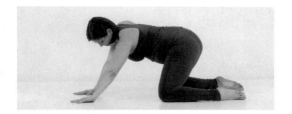

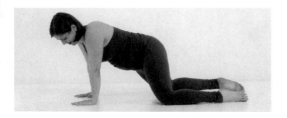

Figure Eights

Remain on your hands and knees. Begin by moving your hips from side to side a few times. Then move into a figure eight pattern: swing your hips to the right, gently tuck your pelvis toward the center of your body, and swing your hips to the other side. Again, find the depth of movement that feels good. Move slowly and feel the stretch through your hips and back, as you bring your awareness to your baby. Your baby will love this movement, as it gently rocks her in your belly. It may feel a little awkward at first, but just keep moving your hips and pelvis until it becomes more instinctual.

BENEFITS: Hip circles and figure eights helps you access your pelvic floor better by taking the weight of your baby off your pelvic floor muscles. The fluid movement improves circulation in the tissues of your lower back, hips, and pelvis.

Jane's Pelvic Toning and Strengthening Advice

- *Do* strengthen the pelvic floor muscles if yours are healthy or low tone.
- *Don't* grip your pelvic muscles; gentle engagement exercises should simply bring awareness to the tissue.
- *Do* relax between repetitions so you don't fatigue the muscles.
- *Don't* continue the strengthening exercise if you can't feel your pelvic floor muscles release after gentle engagement.
- *Do* spend time learning to release and relax, especially if you have high-tone or excessively tight pelvic muscles. Restorative yoga postures like Supta Baddha Konasana (Reclining Bound Angle Pose) are particularly effective.

Strengthening Your Pelvic Floor Muscles

On your hands and knees, close your eyes and visualize your pelvic floor muscles. Keeping your pelvis and spine still, gently engage, lift, and hold your pelvic floor muscles in the following order: first, the muscles around the urethra; next, those around the vagina; and last, those around the anus. Visualize closing and lifting each sphincter. Then (this is very important) completely release from back to front—anus, vagina, urethra.

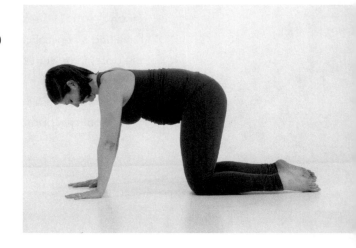

Initially, hold for a short period of time—3 to 5 seconds—and slowly release. *Do not* continue the exercise if you can't feel the muscles release. Gradually build up to holding for 8 to 10 seconds, but don't fatigue the muscles. Rest in Balasana (Child's Pose) between sets—rest and repeat 4 or 5 times. Relaxing between exercises is essential.

Wave Squats

Another effective tool for locating and toning your pelvic floor muscles, this dynamic posture helps bring some awareness to those muscles as you move. You may find this more useful than the longer-held deep squats.

Stand in Tadasana (Mountain Pose) with your feet more than hip-width apart, toes pointing forward. Inhale as you bring your arms over your head; exhale as you come into Utkatasana (Chair Pose). Stick out your bum so you can feel your sitting bones widen behind you, and keep your shin bones as vertical as possible. Inhale again, and as you exhale, tuck your pelvis and place your hands on your thighs; roll up to standing. Repeat this mini vinyasa, following your breath. Inhale to widen your sitting bones as you come down and lengthen the pelvic floor muscles; exhale to tuck your pelvis and lift the muscles as you come back up.

ADVANCED MODIFICATION: Squat a little more deeply, and on the exhalation, take your hands all the way to the floor—or to a block in front of you—before rolling up to standing. If your heels lift off the mat, place a folded blanket or rolled yoga mat under them to stay grounded. Start with 10 to 15 wave squats and work your way up to 20 or 30. These squats should feel good and energizing. If you feel strain in your joints, either go back to the Utkatasana variation or discontinue completely, depending on what your instincts tell you.

CAUTION: This exercise is contraindicated if you have placenta previa or have had a cervical cerclage and are at risk for preterm labor. Discontinue the pose if you start to feel dizzy or nauseous.

BENEFITS: This movement promotes good circulation of the blood and lymphatic fluid in and out of your pelvis. When you do them correctly, Wave Squats support proper function of your pelvic organs.

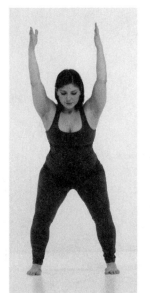
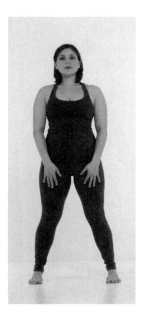
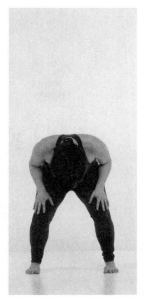
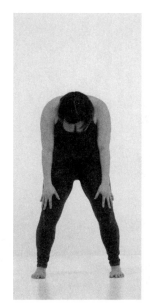

MODIFICATION

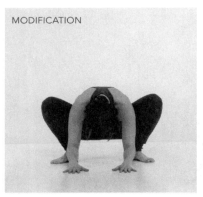
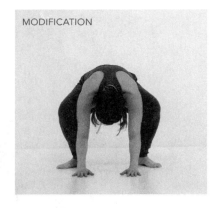

MODIFICATION

MODIFICATION

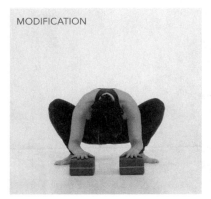
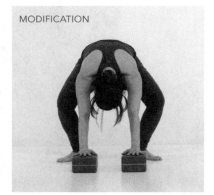

MODIFICATION

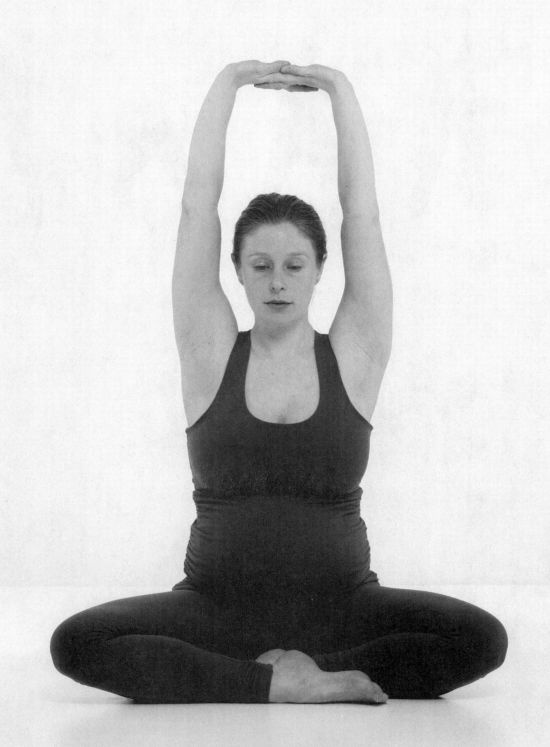

4.

THIRD TRIMESTER

The Home Stretch
From Twenty-Eight to Forty-Two Weeks

Sequences by Margi Young

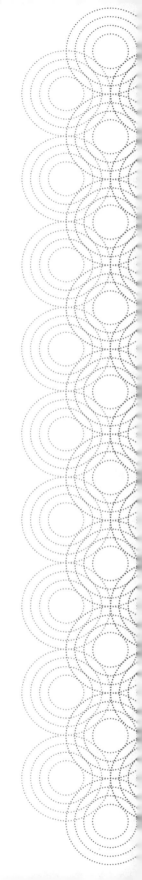

Three more months to go before you can hold your baby in your arms. For some women, the birth will come not a moment too soon—months of raging hormones have brought a litany of aches and pains, emotional upheavals, and a swollen body they barely recognize. For others, pregnancy has been a blessed time of connection (to themselves and to their babies) and of excitement and renewed strength, not to mention great hair and clear skin. But the vast majority of women will probably admit that this journey's been a bit of a mixed bag.

The third trimester can often usher in more of a sense of urgency or impatience than the first two, and it may be difficult to stop yourself from focusing on or even worrying about the future. Luckily, your yoga practice will help ground you both physically and emotionally. The asanas you'll be doing this trimester will no doubt change again as your belly commands more attention and your center of balance shifts.

As ever, so much depends on what's true for you right now. Mary Taylor, the codirector (with her husband, Richard Freeman) of The Yoga Workshop in Boulder, Colorado, practiced advanced series Ashtanga with Pattabhi Jois, her long-time teacher, all the way through her pregnancy. However, my daughter Megan, a yoga practitioner and former professional ballet dancer, found that by her ninth month she could no longer transition easily from one pose to another. She felt uncoordinated and even resentful that her body couldn't do what she wanted it to do.

Suddenly moving from Downward Dog to a lunge became impossible and the source of much frustration. These two examples illustrate that every pregnancy is different. Your practice should uniquely serve your experience and your needs—that's what yoga does. The key is to figure out—by listening, noticing, and exploring—where you are right now (your foundation) and where you need to go (a sense of direction). What do you need today? Do you want to feel more open, get things moving downward, breathe more fully, or stay quiet? Then design your yoga practice accordingly.

The Inside Scoop

Your belly is now front and center. In fact, everything seems to be getting bigger, louder, and more insistent. Your uterus has expanded all the way to your rib cage, where you swear your baby is tap dancing and purposely making it harder for you to breathe. All his kicks, jabs, pokes, and somersaults are your baby's way of responding to your voice, light, or even pain. You've probably gained at least twenty-five to thirty pounds by now, not only because the baby is growing (he'll weigh between six and nine pounds by the time he makes his entrance), but also because you're lugging around a lot of excess baggage: a uterus that has grown to five hundred times its normal size, about eight to ten pounds of placenta, excess blood and amniotic fluid, and an additional two pounds of breast tissue has been loaded onto your frame. So don't be surprised if you feel more tired than usual but also have trouble sleeping and breathing properly. You might even have a little indigestion or heartburn and some swelling in your hands and feet.

As you move into week 37, your baby will begin to drop into position—although that can happen earlier, or not until just before labor starts. This is good news for your rib cage (and your ability to take a full breath), but not for your bladder, which your baby seems to think is a zafu. Expect to be running to the bathroom a lot more frequently. Once he's settled in, he won't have much room to poke and jab, so you'll probably feel more stretches, turns, and wiggles. All through this trimester, you may experience strong intermittent gripping in your belly. These

Braxton-Hicks contractions, or "silent" prelabor cramps, help prepare your uterus for labor by softening your pelvic floor and even dilating your cervix a little—and they do all that painlessly. If you are pregnant for the second or third time, you may experience these contractions more frequently.

Your baby's senses have awakened now—she can see, taste, hear, smell, and respond to your touch. She's perfected the sucking and swallowing actions she'll need to nurse, and her brain has almost fully developed (some researchers even say she now has the ability to remember). She's getting fatter, absorbing antibodies from you that she'll need in the outside world, and her nervous system is just about ready for her debut.

Keep on Moving

Moving your body is as important at this stage of your pregnancy as finding time to reflect deeply and communicate with your baby. Whether you can comfortably and safely keep up a more energizing routine or need to pull way back, a vinyasa yoga practice can still support you, but you may need to broaden the definition of vinyasa a bit. Generally when we hear that word, we think of moving seamlessly from pose to pose on the wave of the breath, much like we do in Ashtanga yoga and the increasingly fast-paced offshoots such as power yoga and prana flow. But nothing in the "rule books" suggests that vinyasa flow needs to be done a particular way. If you need to exhale from Downward Dog to your hands and knees, bring your hands to blocks, then step forward into a lunge slowly and deliberately, that's your new vinyasa sequence.

So while the beauty of vinyasa lies in the way it connects poses—allowing us to come into a pose, settle there (for a breath or two), move out of it, and welcome another one rising up to take its place—this movement also exists within a single pose on a microlevel. On some days, you may want to move into Virabhadrasana II (Warrior II Pose) from Tadasana (Mountain Pose), for example, paying attention to the placement of your feet, arms, and belly as well as the sensations you feel and the trajectory of your thoughts, and then sustain the pose for a few smooth, long breaths—or maybe only one breath. Then you can consciously come out of the pose, taking stock of its effects before deciding how or whether to move into the next asana. On other occasions, you may feel more comfortable coming in and out of Virabhadrasana II a few times, letting your breath (and your ability to balance) dictate the pace. If you feel particularly tired or your balance is off, you can borrow a trick from Iyengar yoga and use a chair, resting the thigh of your bent leg on the chair seat.

Nourishing the Koshas

Vinyasa's notion of impermanence—"this too shall pass" being the operative phrase in your third trimester—reminds us that things arise, they abide, and they dissolve both on and off the mat. Every moment, thought, or action that arises is all there is for that moment; it then dissolves as a new moment, thought, or action surfaces. Remembering the beauty and flow of such impermanence will serve you well during this trimester, especially toward the end when you may feel uncomfortable and heavy and afraid you'll never get your body back. Embrace "this too shall pass" during labor and birthing—and parenting, too. Those intense labor pains? Each one arises, abides with intensity and purpose, and then thankfully dissolves, moving your baby closer to birth.

Vinyasa's literal translation, "placing in a special way," means much more than how we sequence a Sun Salutation. It requires us to place *everything* in a special way: our feet, arms, shoulders, neck, and hips; the body as a whole; our breath, mind, and heart. In other words, a vinyasa practice is the practice of paying attention with all our senses as things arise, abide, and dissolve, actively engaging all the koshas (the five "layers" of the body) in our quest for self-awareness both on and off the mat. Bringing this understanding to your pregnancy, you can place your attention on how your body feels; what it needs; and how your actions, words, emotions, and thoughts affect your baby and your experience.

The first layer (the *annamaya kosha*) is the physical body, what you can touch, see, and move. As you move closer to the end of your pregnancy, how your body feels takes on a new level of importance.

You are paying attention not only to your own physical sensations but your baby's response to those sensations. Notice your posture, your body's alignment. What does your body need in each pose to create more space, more joy, and more connection? The ancients referred to this kosha as the "food body," a translation that lends itself well to metaphors. What do you need to do to nourish yourself? To prepare for the birth of your baby? This applies to foods, for sure, but also to what thoughts feed your confidence and which ones restrict it or feed your fears.

Once you take an inventory of the physical sensations in your body, begin focusing on your "breath body" (the *pranamaya kosha*). Sit or lie still and feel the movement of prana throughout your body. Notice the beating of your baby's heart, of your own heart. Don't try to control or change anything at first; simply observe the rhythm and texture of your breath. Where does the inhalation begin and the exhalation end? Does your breathing feel smooth or jagged? As feelings surface, do they affect the evenness of your breath? Once you know the quality of your breathing, you can begin to move it through your body more easily. During your asana practice, using Ujjayi Pranayama (Victorious Breath) will help you monitor the intensity of your vinyasa and keep it at a level that's appropriate for your body's needs and limitations right now. Consciously directing your breath into your womb will help you listen to and communicate with your baby.

The third subtle body layer, the *manomaya kosha* (the thinking mind), needs little introduction. You probably already know how the activities of your mind can influence your body, send your emotions in a million different directions, and make breathing a challenge. The sheath of the mind also governs the nervous system. When your mind is agitated it affects your nervous system—causing you to feel restless, anxious, or fearful—and the rest of the physical body, too. Conversely, as you steady your breath, your mind settles, your nerves calm down, and your body feels more open, maybe a little freer. So use the breath as a bridge between your body and your mind. Every inhalation gathers your inner resources (your breath and your mind); each exhalation moves them into your body, releasing any physical tightness or emotional sensations that get lodged in your joints and muscles. Practicing the quieting of your mind will help you immensely during labor and birthing. But don't wait until you're in active labor to remember the connection!

As you feel more at home in your growing body and find a breathing rhythm that works for you, you may notice a deeper level of awareness; that's the *vijnanamaya kosha* in action—your wisdom or "discerning mind." I think of it as the inherent intelligence of the body that we access and learn to trust through our yoga practice. *Vijnanamaya* moments allow you to see into the truth of your experience and know you have what it takes to move through these last few months and birth your baby in the way he is supposed to be born. The discerning mind doesn't judge; it simply notices with loving curiosity and affection.

You may have experienced a taste of the *anandamaya kosha*, the "bliss body," in yoga class. Perhaps there's a moment when you move into a pose and everything just comes together. You aren't thinking about the how, where, and what; everything (your posture, your breath, and your mind) is aligned, and your body simply opens and receives. At that moment, you stop practicing and start doing. When you as witness are no longer separate from your experience, when you allow your whole being to join together with your baby to usher her into the world, and when you feel as though you two are one, you have glimpsed the anandamaya kosha—the body of pure bliss.

Eating for Vitality

Ideally, you've eaten a healthy diet throughout your pregnancy—except for indulging some late-night cravings. The third trimester should be no different. In fact, now is the time to eat plenty of immunity-boosting foods because, according to Western medicine, this trimester is when a mother passes her own antibodies to her baby through the placenta. Your baby's immune system won't be fully developed until after he is born. Ayurvedic medicine agrees, although the ancient texts have a different way of describing what happens. They say that, beginning in the eighth month, the mother passes her *ojas* (vitality, vigor) along to the baby, and that handoff can take about a month to complete. The sages say that the purest ojas resides in the mother's heart and nourishes the subtle energies in the body, which in turn feed the body's vigor, vitality, and immunity. An abundance of this vital essence—minute portions of which get released in our blood, muscles, fat, bones, nervous system, reproductive fluid, and heart—ensures good health; depletion brings on disease or chronic conditions. The handoff of antibodies, or ojas, gives the baby a healthy head start as he positions himself to leave the womb and enter the world.

Ayurveda also says that the mother's transferred ojas imbues the baby with his own consciousness, separate from the mother's, which prepares him for life outside the womb. Ayurveda encourages a mother to meditate often and visualize her baby as distinct from herself. Creating a practice around that may help you build a healthy relationship with your baby before he's even born, a relationship that will continue to strengthen throughout your life together. In a very practical sense, beginning this physical and emotional separation can also help you release your pelvic floor and usher your baby out more quickly and (hopefully) less painfully. Giving birth is ishvara pranidhana in action—quite literally, surrendering the fruits of your labor.

Nourishing the Soul

As we know, we take more than just food into our bodies as nourishment. As pregnant women, we need to be even more mindful of what impressions we absorb—sights, sounds, tastes, reactions, feelings—and what we pass along to our baby. Once we've built superior ojas and a strong immune system, we need to create a supportive environment that encourages less stress and more nurturing, caring, and immunity-building activities. To do that, ayurvedic practitioners, like my friend Kathryn Templeton, recommend focusing on gratitude, sleep, and connection.

GRATITUDE

Before you even get out of bed in the morning (and again before you drop off to sleep at night), spend a few moments affirming your appreciation and gratitude for your pregnancy, for your family and others who support you, and for your baby. Prayer, meditation, and affirmations are all important to cultivate and support ojas.

SLEEP

Good-quality sleep should be on your ojas-support list. For most women, sleep is elusive in the third trimester, so it's hard to figure out how to get any at all, let alone the high-quality variety. If that's your experience, practice Yoga Nidra—the deeply restorative practice of a "yoga nap"—either in the morning or in the late afternoon; practicing too close to bedtime may confuse your body into thinking it's already rested and ready for a new day!

CONNECTIONS

Being with friends, laughing, taking walks in nature, continuing to do what you love—all of these activities build strong immunity. Sharing joys as well as worries, laughter as well as tears with other pregnant women and your partner will lift your spirits, allay your fears, and increase the vital essence you are now passing along to your baby.

Your Yoga Practice

By the third trimester, you can keep frustrations to a minimum by coming to practice with no preconceived notion of what that practice should or shouldn't look like. When San Francisco OM teacher Margi Young could no longer lie on her belly, twist, or even step forward in ways that were familiar to her, she discovered a whole new awareness. "Suddenly there was so much more to observe, and I could depend on every day being vastly different from the one before," she says. "I just needed to remind myself of the Buddha's brilliant dissertation on impermanence. It is only for this short time that Bow Pose will not be part of my life."

So what part of your familiar yoga practice *can* be part of your life? Like everything else in pregnancy, it depends. You'll want to take into account what feels good to your body, what nourishes and supports your baby, and what you did on your mat prior to becoming pregnant.

Creating space in your body and moving the energy downward will probably make the most sense now. A practice that includes the full range of motion may help counter fatigue, listlessness, or any anxiety that's been building up. Think again of yoga as a good training ground for labor, birthing, and even parenthood. By placing your attention on all the koshas, your practice will help you build strength, staying power, and flexibility—both physically and mentally. It will give you a deeper connection to your breath, help you ride (and rein in) the potentially wide-ranging fluctuations of your mind, and trust in the power of your intuition. Just remember that your balance—and quite likely your energy levels—will be different, so give yourself permission to modify on the fly. Keep a collection of props at the ready: a couple of blocks to rest your hands on; a bolster to relax into; and two blankets to sit on. Then position yourself near a wall, just in case.

STANDING POSES

Although it may seem impossible right now, directing your attention to your feet will help ground you physically and energetically. Standing poses can also invigorate a sagging posture by elongating and strengthening your spine, which currently has a heavier load to bear, and releasing and relaxing your shoulders and neck. I like to think of standing poses as "fake-it-till-you-make-it" postures; standing tall and strong actually helps you *feel* strong and capable. And you'll certainly need that going through labor. Poses like Tadasana (Mountain Pose), Urdhva Hastasana (Upward Salute), and Virabhadrasana I (Warrior I Pose) can lift your diaphragm off your protruding belly, giving you a little more breathing room and, as an added bonus, strengthening your resolve. Emotionally as well as physically, standing poses increase your willpower, determination, and stamina.

MODIFICATIONS: If you feel tired, position yourself against a wall; in fact, allow the wall to *be* the back of your body instead of falling into it when you get tired. Don't stay in standing poses longer than is comfortable (10 to 20 seconds should be fine), and come out slowly and deliberately as you move to the next pose.

STANDING FORWARD EXTENSIONS

Your standing forward bends may not feel that great anymore, with your belly so far out in front of you. That doesn't mean you have to give them up, but it does mean you should approach them in a way that's more comfortable for you and doesn't put pressure on your baby. To enjoy the benefits of forward bends more safely, extend your spine instead of rounding your back over your legs; bend from your hips instead of your waist. This elongation will release any tightness in your hamstrings and your lower back and increase circulation to your legs, kidneys, and pelvis. It will also create space in your belly and allow your pelvic floor muscles to soften and spread. These poses continue the strengthening and elongating work of your standing poses, increasing your energy, realigning your spine, and toning your vaginal and cervical walls.

MODIFICATIONS: Keep your feet at least hip-width apart in Uttanasana (Standing Forward Bend). Place your hands on blocks positioned far enough in front of you so you can elongate your spine and lengthen the front of your body. An overwhelming favorite of third-trimester women, Prasarita Padottanasana (Wide-Legged Standing Forward Bend) can be done resting your hands on a chair seat if touching the floor seems impossible right now. If you experience any pressure or discomfort in your pelvic floor, narrow your stance until you feel more comfortable.

BACKBENDS

There's much to love about backbends, especially when you've grown weary of your baby's weight bearing down on your kidneys and bladder. The litany of benefits to enjoy from backbends in the third trimester is pretty impressive. These poses stretch and tone the front of your body, which has worked hard all these months to hold itself up and accommodate your expanding uterus. They increase circulation in your upper body, as well as in your kidneys, pelvis, and uterus. They can lift your spirits and give you a wonderful sense of accomplishment. They can even reduce water retention—an uncomfortable side effect of pregnancy for a lot of women. While natural backbenders may feel comfortable continuing to practice Urdhva Dhanurasana (Upward-Facing Bow Pose) safely in their third trimester, others find unsupported backbends too aggressive. Luckily, you can reap all the benefits of bending backward without having to commit to a daily practice of Wheel Pose. Supported but energizing backbends like Ustrasana (Camel Pose) with your hands on blocks or your head against the wall or completely passive ones like Supta Baddha Konasana (Reclining Bound Angle Pose) or Supta Virasana (Reclining Hero Pose) work just as well.

CAUTION: Unsupported backbends with a very pregnant belly can pull on your already vulnerable abdominal muscles, which may prove to be too much of a strain. Remember that the hormone relaxin has already compromised the smooth muscles of your uterus, so guard against overstretching.

SEATED FORWARD BENDS

Much like standing forward bends and extensions, this group of poses can release stiffness in your lower back and strengthen your spine. Poses like Baddha Konasana (Bound Angle Pose) and Upavistha Konasana (Wide-Angle Seated Pose) can also relieve pressure around your pubic bone by slightly lifting the weight of your uterus off your pelvic floor. Done correctly, they can also tone, stretch, and soften your pelvic floor muscles and your vaginal opening—great preparation for labor and birthing. However, if you can't bend forward without rounding your spine or collapsing the front of your body (thereby compromising your ability to breathe), then reach forward from your hips and extend your spine instead. Your focus should be on lifting your chest, making lots of space in your belly, and moving your ribs away from your hips. Seated extensions like Balasana (Child's Pose) with knees

Forward Bending after Twenty Weeks

De West, a pre- and postnatal teacher in Boulder, Colorado, discourages her pregnant students from doing any forward bending after about twenty weeks, preferring to teach the upright version of all seated poses. "I find that in about 85 percent of the mothers, just sitting upright is enough to stretch their hamstrings, open their spine, and make room for the baby," she says. Most pregnant women can't bend forward without rounding their spine or shortening the pubis-to-sternum area, which compresses the womb. Listening to your body and moving consciously will dictate how much you round or how far you extend. Always err on the side of comfort and visualize how your baby is receiving each pose.

wide apart or Uttana Shishosana (Extended Puppy Pose) have a quieting, grounding effect on your nervous system.

MODIFICATIONS: In Upavistha Konasana or any wide-legged seated forward bend, stay more upright, which will help lift the weight of your uterus, and keep your legs a comfortable distance apart. Spreading your pubic bones too wide, coupled with the weight of your uterus, may cause sheering in your pelvis. As an end-of-the-day treat, extend over bolsters or blankets for a more restorative (and more comfortable) Balasana.

TWISTS

One goal of prenatal yoga is to create space and to find a balance between effort and ease, strength and receptivity, and lift and release. Twists get rid of stiffness in your lower back, keep your spine strong and flexible, and increase blood flow to your reproductive organs and adrenal glands. But like any pose, twists create problems if you get too aggressive or overenthusiastic.

During pregnancy, it's best to avoid twisting poses that create a squeezing sensation in your abdomen or pelvis. But don't cross all twists off your list. Bharadvajasana (Simple Seated Twist Pose) and other open-belly twists feel wonderful, especially on your lower back, upper back, and shoulders. They will keep your shoulders, upper back, and neck flexible, which will make nursing and carrying your baby a whole lot more comfortable. Once you've gone past your due date, a yoga-savvy midwife or doula may recommend closed twists that cue your body to squeeze and release, but just to be safe, ask before you do any on your own.

MODIFICATIONS: If you feel your posture sagging, sit about 6 inches to a foot away from the wall. Twist toward—and place your hands on—the wall to get a nice lift in your spine and a sense of spaciousness in your belly.

INVERSIONS

If you've always loved inversions, and you've made standing on your head part of your regular practice, there's no reason to stop doing it as long as it still feels good. Many women shelve unsupported inversions around the sixth month; others keep going until about the eighth month.

Inversions do a lot of things: release tension in your neck, shoulders, and upper back; energize your endocrine system; and even help lessen water retention. But the main reason many women continue doing them is that turning upside down lifts the baby off the pelvis for what can be a blissful few moments of relief from the achiness and heaviness pregnant mamas feel. And who wouldn't benefit from the boost of energy that inversions provide? Even if you're part of the die-hard upside-down club, however, inverting may not make much sense by the time you reach the middle or end of your eighth month. By then your body is ready to focus on the apana vayu, the downward-moving flow of energy, encouraging your baby to begin her descent into the pelvis in preparation for birth. Going upside down could work against that.

MODIFICATIONS: If you do practice Sirasasana (Headstand), Adho Mukha Vrksasana (Handstand), or any other inversion, be safe and use the wall. Better yet, lift up at the corner where two walls intersect, placing one foot on each wall.

SQUATTING

By now you're probably an old pro at squats if you've been practicing them for the last several months of your pregnancy. Keep on keepin' on, because squatting will help you widen your sitting bones and lengthen and soften your pelvic floor muscles—good things to do in preparation for labor and birthing. Make sure to keep your spine long and your sacrum either in a neutral position or tilted slightly forward when you squat. Avoid rounding your back, which narrows the pelvic opening and makes it difficult for your baby's head to settle into position properly. If squatting is difficult or tiring, stand with your back against the wall and only go down as far as you can while maintaining good pelvic alignment.

MODIFICATIONS: Place a block or two a few inches away from the wall to squat on. Alternatively, come in and out of the squat several times before settling onto your support. You can also lean forward slightly from your hip joints as long as you can keep your sitting bones on the wall.

CAUTION: Don't do deep squats late in your pregnancy if your baby is not facing the right way (that is, with her head down and facing your back). Deep squatting encourages the baby to drop farther down into your pelvis, and if she settles in the wrong position, she'll have trouble turning the right way.

PRANAYAMA

You've probably also kept up with your pranayama practice throughout your pregnancy. But if not, the third trimester is a good time to return to it and reacquaint yourself with techniques that can help you breathe consciously and lovingly. You want your relationship to your breath to be second nature by the time your labor starts. By incorporating pranayama into your daily routine (and practicing it often throughout the day), your breath will become a valuable ally and resource all through your labor. Ujjayi Pranayama (Victorious Breath) helps keep the inhalation and exhalation long and smooth. Viloma Pranayama I (Interval Breathing I), with a three-part inhalation and a slow, smooth exhalation, can be particularly helpful to quell anxiety and soften the pains during transition. To practice it, inhale the breath up to your navel and pause; inhale up to your rib cage and pause; then inhale all the way up to your collarbones, pause; and exhale completely, long and slow.

MODIFICATIONS: Do not retain your breath in prenatal pranayama. It's fine, of course, to inhale and pause, exhale and pause, but do not grab onto the breath and hold it. Retaining your breath exerts pressure on your abdomen—which is never a good idea when you're pregnant.

Third-Trimester Challenges

For some women, the third trimester feels much longer than three months—those last few weeks can drag on forever, especially if your baby seems to be taking her time exiting the womb. Physically your body is under a great deal of strain carting around more weight than it's used to. If you have old hip or back injuries, they may resurface, mainly because hormones have made your joints relatively unstable. Since the hormone relaxin, which widens the pelvis during labor and birthing, doesn't confine its effects to the pelvic region, women who already have hypermobile joints may experience instability and aches and pains; most women complain about at least a little joint pain, as well as constipation and even heartburn. Make sure you pay close attention to how poses feel on your pelvic outlet, groin, hips, and sacrum. If you feel any pressure at all, pull back. Do not overstretch!

Many women, whether they're hyper-flexible or uber-stiff, suffer back pain at some point during their pregnancies. Once again, you can blame relaxin, which makes it a challenge for the ligaments in the lower back to counter the weight of a protruding belly. And the abdominals are already taxed so they can't offer much help. Do whatever you can to support your lower back. Warm compresses on your sacrum can help. Squats or an upright Upavistha Konasana (Wide-Angle Seated Pose) or Baddha Konasana (Bound Angle Pose) against the wall can strengthen your back. Restorative poses like a bolster-intensive Balasana (Child's Pose) can relax and relieve tired muscles. The bonus? These poses also release tension in your hip joints and groin, create space for your baby, and gently encourage your pelvis to open.

Swelling in your hands and feet can also be an uncomfortable side effect of your third trimester. As long as the swelling doesn't come on suddenly and settle in your hands or face (a sign of pregnancy-induced hypertension), this side effect is more of an annoyance than a cause of concern. Luckily, inverted yoga poses like Viparita Karani (Legs-Up-the-Wall Pose) can reduce the swelling. Just make sure to place a bolster or a couple of rolled blankets under your sacrum so it is higher than your heart. Opt for anything that can cool you down—cool drinks of water, a cool or tepid bath, and plenty of watery fruits and vegetables. Yoga poses in which you rest your head on something (a bolster, blanket, chair, or your arms) are also cooling.

Viparita Karani and other supported inversions can also help minimize varicose veins and maybe even hemorrhoids (which are really varicose veins of the rectum)—both caused by hormones, of course, and increased blood flow—by taking the pressure off the legs and the pelvic floor. Some yoga-savvy midwives discourage lying on your back for any length of time at the end of your pregnancy—even in Viparita Karani with your sacrum lifted on a bolster—because that may encourage your baby to rest his spine against your back, a less-than-optimal position that can make the birthing experience more difficult for him and for you. If you're not sure of your baby's position, check with your midwife first or shelve this pose until after your baby is born.

The position of your baby makes a difference in what you experience during this trimester. If you're "carrying high," that is, if your baby hasn't dropped into position yet, heartburn may suddenly (or once again) become a nagging presence. Inversions won't work that well for you; you don't want to encourage the baby to move farther up. So you probably should shelve the upside-down poses such as Adho Mukha Svanasana (Downward-Facing Dog Pose), Sirsasana (Headstand), and Adho Mukha Vrksasana (Handstand), if you're still doing them, and focus on poses that give you as much space as you can get between your diaphragm and your baby. A well-lifted and supported Supta Baddha Konasana (Reclining Bound Angle Pose) or Supta Virasana (Reclining Hero Pose) should do the trick; so will Virabhadrasana I (Warrior I Pose)

Megan's Story

All through my pregnancy, I felt deeply connected to my body, yet toward the end, I began to resent it. I felt as though I had no control over my body, and I hated the fact that I couldn't use it in ways I was used to. By the end of my pregnancy, I had nested about as much as I could stand, and all I could do was wait. But waiting was rough. It made me impatient and more irritated about my condition. So I turned to yoga. Pranayama, in particular, made me feel less out of control and set me up to trust in the power of my own breath. My asana practice, even though it had changed, reminded me that I was strong, that I could balance, and it gave me opportunities to practice letting go. It was hard for me to admit that I couldn't possibly control everything. So I welcomed other women's birth stories, read books, gathered anything that would help me steer the ship and be prepared. Reading and sharing stories and information gave me control over something—my own preparations.

with your arms over your head. Also, see Melissa's Sequence for Indigestion on page 52.

If your baby has already begun her descent, you will probably feel a lot of discomfort and pressure bearing down on your cervix and bladder. Mild and supported inversions and backbends should bring some temporary relief.

Fatigue and listlessness, common complaints toward the end of pregnancy, can literally and figuratively weigh you down. That's why most women like to include active poses in their daily practice along with the restoratives. My daughter Megan said getting up and moving helped her morale, took her mind off the waiting game, and even tempered her impatience. Techniques like Viloma Pranayama (Interval Breathing), with the three-part breath focused on the inhalation, can also lift your spirits.

Managing Fear and Anxiety

Along with all the excitement and joyous anticipation, you may also experience some anxiety in the last trimester, which is quite normal. In fact, in *Birthing from Within*, Pam England says, "Worry is the work of pregnancy." That didn't make sense to me at first. If we stay true to our practice, communicate with our baby, and prepare for this experience as best we can, why would we need to worry? Because worry is what the mind does, rationally or irrationally. England says that we must all face our fears, and acknowledge them out loud, before we can let them go.

When I was pregnant with my first daughter, I had plenty of fears: *What if my baby dies in childbirth? What if I die in childbirth? What if I can't handle a no-drug-zone birth? What if I don't love my baby?* Never once did I give voice to any of them. I was afraid that by saying something I would make it come true. Looking back, I wish I had connected with other women who were pregnant. It would have helped me realize that all women have some fear around giving birth and it wasn't just me.

Holding on to fear and anxiety can do more than make your pregnancy miserable; it can also impinge on your ability to have a smooth labor and birthing experience. Remember that pregnancy brings with it loads of friendly hormones to ensure that your body can provide optimal nourishment (both physically and emotionally) and a healthy environment for your baby, as well as a safe passageway into the world. But when you are stressed, anxious, and fearful, your body perceives that you are in danger and virtually suspends its prenatal hormonal activity. It instead mobilizes its fight-or-flight resources, which include pouring stress hormones (like adrenaline, catecholamine, and cortisol) into your bloodstream so you can react appropriately, and it instructs all "nonessential" systems (like the reproductive, immune, and digestive systems) to slow down and wait out the danger. According to an article in the *Journal of Perinatal Education*, the hormones that allow women to give birth and nurse effectively "are all easily 'disturbed.'" In other words, if a woman feels threatened, fearful, or anxious, the levels of stress hormones will prevent her labor from beginning (or continuing). One early study (1987) on pregnant lab mice showed that when the mice were disturbed, especially by a lack of privacy, surges of the stress hormone catecholamine halted early labor. This was nature's way of responding "to threats, potential or real, in the birth environment, protecting the mother and her young." While you may not have actual predators ready to pounce, your inability to let go of stress or face your fears can cause you problems.

HOW TO ALLAY YOUR FEARS

No matter what anxieties you face, coming back to your yoga practice can prevent you from turning into a ball of fear. Just being on your mat and exploring a few poses will get you out of your head and into your body, which will have a calming effect on your nervous system and rein in your imagination. Don't count on restorative poses to soothe your nerves; after all, lying still in a dark room may make your mind race even more! Get moving, if you can. Do poses (against the wall, if you prefer) that build strength and resolve. Once again, standing poses like Utthita Trikonasana (Extended Triangle Pose) and Virabhdrasana (Warrior Pose) can give you a sense of being in control. Stay connected to your breath by adding a chant or mantra to any breathing practice (like the Rose Petal Breath on the next page), which may also assuage your fears.

Hiring a midwife or doula to partner with you as you transition toward giving birth can calm a lot of the anxieties you may feel about the process. By now, you've no doubt chosen your birthing team, but just in case you haven't, it bears repeating that midwife- or doula-assisted birthing experiences result in far fewer medical interventions. These supporters act as intermediaries for you, letting your wishes be known and running interference for you so you can stay internal and focus on allowing your body to prepare for and open to the birth of your child.

The Rose Petal Breath

Jane Austin uses this lovely practice as a way of releasing fears and doubts.

Sitting comfortably—with your back against a wall, if you wish—spend a few minutes noticing your breathing. Feel the air entering and filling up your lungs as you inhale; allow the breath to release completely as you exhale. Now bring your attention to your mouth and moisten your lips with your tongue. Separate your lips very slightly as if holding a rose petal between them, allowing them to get really soft. Breathe in through your nose and out through your gently parted lips. With each breath you take, soften all the muscles of your face. As you continue to breathe, be reminded of the link between the muscles of your mouth and jaw and those deep within your pelvis. As you soften your face, you may experience the release of any tension, gripping, or holding in the muscles of your hips and pelvis. Ultimately, this softness in the tissue will create more space for your baby to move through your body. With each inhalation, say one of the following aspirations to yourself,

I have all that I need to birth my baby.
I have all that I need to mother my baby.
I am all that I need to be to mother my baby.

With each exhalation, say the following to yourself,

I let go of doubt or fear.

COMMUNITY

Signing up for a prenatal class, even this far along in your pregnancy, will connect you with other women on the path and may help you put your fears in perspective. In some respects, prenatal yoga gives you permission to be supported—physically with props and emotionally by sharing your experiences and concerns and listening to others tell their stories—and to realize that your fears are universal.

MEDITATION

Patanjali's Yoga Sutra (II.33) asks us to cultivate the opposite attitude as a way of diffusing a strong emotion or a destructive, persistent thought. If you feel scared or anxious, spend some time visualizing your strength, feeling joyful anticipation, and acknowledging your innate ability to create life. Allow your mind to move into your belly and send soothing, full breaths to your baby.

All of these suggestions—getting on your mat, reaching out to other women, and sitting in meditation—are variations of *abhyasa* (diligent, persistent practice) and *vairagya* (letting go). Abhyasa is the subtle effort we need to bring our mind back to the present moment and not allow it to run amok; vairagya is what helps us release the grip of whatever has a hold on us. According to Chip Hartranft in his commentary on the Yoga Sutra, vairagya means "not getting stirred up." In other words, can you notice something as it presents itself (abhyasa) and not react to it (vairagya)? Try sitting with your thoughts and projections and noticing them as though you were an impartial observer. See yourself reacting as those thoughts come to the surface. Can you set aside the story you tell yourself (the reasons for your fears) and direct your attention to any sensations in your body that these feelings create? Allow an exhalation to soften and release the tightness in the muscles in which those sensations have settled.

Doing all that, of course, takes determination (tapas), self-reflection (svadhyaya), and surrender (ishvara pranidhana), all of which we practice on our yoga mat all the time. When we have the courage and willpower to name our fears and see them as traps set by the mind and imagination, that's tapas. When we can notice our traps without judgment, bringing a sense of friendliness and tenderness to that part of ourselves, that's svadhyaya. And when we can make friends with those fears—*Ah yes, so it's you again. Let me look at you*—even for a breath or two, we can more easily set them aside. That's ishvara pranidhana, the act of surrender, which frees our mind to see the divinity in all beings, including ourselves, and reminds us that we are exactly who and where we need to be to give birth and mother our baby. If all that feels overwhelming, just remember that whenever you're on your mat, yoga asks you to practice diligently, listen intently to your body's response, and stay open to the outcome—without trying to control, judge, or filter it through someone else's experiences.

> ### Tips to Calm a Racing Mind
>
> • Do something physical to move the stress from your mind into your body from which it can be released.
> • Spend time meditating to further center your mind in the present moment.
> • Put on some soothing music (or chanting), sit back against a propped-up bolster or in your favorite chair, and rub your belly with some gently heated sesame or almond oil. Focus on creating a joyful connection between you and your baby.
> • Talk or sing to your baby; tell him you're honored to be his mother and you're eagerly awaiting his arrival.

Assessing Your Baby's Position

Toward the end of your third trimester, your baby will begin to enter the birth canal in one of several positions. Although it's sometimes difficult to tell, the more you get to know what your baby feels like, the easier it'll be to know what position she's in. Most babies move around and don't start to settle into birthing position until between week 32 and week 35, so if her feet seem to be pressing down on your pubic bone before then, you probably don't need to be concerned. Most midwives say many babies don't commit to a position until week 37.

For the smoothest birth experience, for both you and your baby, your baby's head should be down and her chin tucked slightly so that the softest, smallest part of her head will press against your cervix to open it. For that to happen, she must face your back, and her back should face forward. This position is called the occiput anterior (OA). Almost as ideal a position is if the baby has her back turned slightly to the right (ROA) or the left (LOA).

With her head down and her back facing yours, your baby is in an occiput posterior (OP) position. Instead of the soft part of her head bearing down and opening your cervix, it might be her forehead, which is wider and harder. If you can't tell if she's posterior before you go into labor, you no doubt will know once it starts. Intense back labor is usually your first clue—the baby's back is pressing against your sacrum. Her head is also pressing against your bladder, so you may feel the urge to urinate after each contraction. Unfortunately, because the baby's head isn't in the right position, your labor will usually take longer and be less productive. Just like with OA, your baby's back can be slightly off to the right or left in the posterior position.

When your baby is in the occiput transverse (OT) position, although her head is still down where it should be, her back is facing your side instead of your front. Just like a posterior position, her head isn't aligned optimally with your cervix, making labor and birth more challenging.

BREECH

Most women are familiar with breech birth, which often sounds the cesarean alarm among OB/GYNs. Breech babies can be headed down the birth canal feet first, bottom first, or even with their legs crossed like little yogis. If your baby is in this position, don't panic. Many midwives have lots of tricks up their sleeves for righting the ship, so to speak.

If your baby is posterior or transverse, don't do poses that would encourage him to rest his back against yours. Forgo supine poses like Supta Baddha Konasana (Reclining Bound Angle Pose), Supta Virasana (Reclining Hero Pose), or even Viparita Karani (Legs-Up-the-Wall Pose) during the last four weeks or so of pregnancy, unless your baby is already in the optimal OA position. Avoid deep squats as well. Squatting opens the pelvic outlet and encourages the baby down into the birth canal, which is great if he's in the right position but not so good if he isn't.

Your Yoga Practice

Your midwife or doula will probably have plenty of ways to help guide your baby into the right position, including yoga poses, acupuncture, swimming, and hypnosis. If your baby is already in there, keep doing whatever you've been doing, including squats, to move him farther down into the birth canal. Otherwise, focus on belly-down poses that will align, open, and release your pelvic floor muscles and ligaments. Spend time in meditation and restorative poses to lower your stress level, which could be contributing to an overly constricted pelvic floor. Some experts suggest that when the pelvic floor muscles are either too tight or misaligned, there isn't enough room for the baby to settle in comfortably. Pelvic floor sequences like those in Chapter 3 may help.

VISUALIZE

Spending time in reflection toward the end of this trimester with your hands on your belly, feeling your baby's movements and visualizing how she's taking up space there, will give you a good indication of where she's headed. Can you feel her head or her bottom, her shoulder or the roundness of her back? When she pokes and jabs, where do you feel it? If her feet kick your belly, she's probably posterior, which isn't ideal. Side jabs generally mean she's in the correct position.

To help encourage your baby to shift, try hands-and-knees poses in which your sitting bones are higher than your head, especially if your baby is breech. These include Adho Mukha Svanasana (Downward-Facing Dog Pose) and Uttana Shishosana (Extended Puppy Pose). If you already have a strong inversion practice, try Ardha Adho Mukha Vrksasana (Half Handstand) at the wall. All of these poses encourage your baby to move away from your pelvic outlet and reposition herself correctly. You'll need to stay in Uttana Shishosana for at least 30 to 45 minutes to release and open your pelvis enough. Another particularly useful upside-down pose is what Gail Tully of Spinning Babies calls the Forward-Leaning Inversion, which she says can release the uterosacral ligament and give your baby extra room to maneuver. This pose can work well if your baby is breech, lying posteriorly, or if you're having twins. Spinningbabies.com provides complete instructions for you and your partner.

LISTENING AND RELEASING: YOUR THIRD TRIMESTER PRACTICE

MARGI YOUNG

Throughout your practice today, bring your attention to your uterus, your belly, and your baby, setting an intention to notice any new sensations as they present themselves. Make this a time to listen deeply to what your body and your baby need, and respond accordingly. When your mind wanders, let your baby bring you back. Every time you practice this sequence, it will be a new adventure. Some days, you may feel like moving through the sequence vinyasa-style. Other days, you may want to linger in one of the more restorative poses or spend the time singing to your baby.

Connection

Sit in a comfortable position and close your eyes. If you need a little extra support, place your back against a wall, sliding your sitting bones as close as possible to the wall so your spine is vertical. Soften into your experience and resist any inclination to force or push. Gently set aside the ten thousand things on your to-do list and ease into a state of being right here. If demands resurface, simply observe them and then let them go. Remember, you are creating a precious human life, and the cultivation of mindful softness and ease is crucial for both of you.

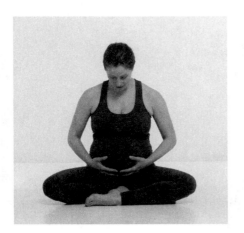

Rest your hands on your belly and let your attention settle onto your baby. Notice any sensations: movement, stillness, joy, numbness, fear, pain—anything. Now is not the time to analyze; just witness and watch with a sense of curiosity and acceptance.

Meditation

Now start to deepen your breath. For 5 breaths, feel both lungs inflate and open on your inhalation and soften and deflate on your exhalation. For the next 5 breaths, imagine that your baby is riding the wavelike movement of your breath.

Chanting

Begin the sweet ritual of singing to your baby. You can chant OM—or anything you wish. Sing a lullaby or a favorite song; short of extreme heavy metal, nothing is off limits. Instead of projecting your voice outward, sing softly and feel that the soothing tones are strengthening the bond between you and your baby.

Pranayama

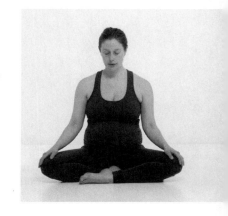

Use the power of your breath to connect to your pelvic floor. Close your eyes and begin breathing in and out through your nose. When you're ready, inhale to a count of 3, 4, or 5 and allow your pelvic floor muscles to release downward. As you exhale, allow your pelvic floor to lift gently. Make the exhalation at least the same length as the inhalation but preferably a couple of counts longer. Release any gripping in your belly. Repeat 10 times.

MODIFICATION: If you have trouble making your exhalation long and smooth, relax your mouth completely and exhale through your gently parted lips. (See the Rose Petal Breath on page 117.)

Seated Warm-ups

From your comfortable seated position, interlace your fingers and reach your arms up to the sky. Be aware of the length you are creating through your belly, as well as the breadth through your back. Now place your right hand on the floor by your right hip and enjoy a side bend to the right, resting your left hand behind your head. Feel as if you are loosening any rigidity around your baby. Remain here for 3 full breaths. Come back to center and repeat on the left side. Do each side 3 times.

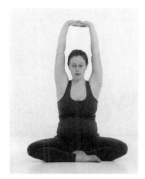 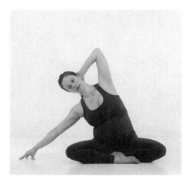 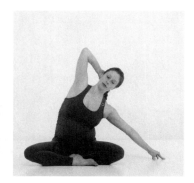

Marjaryasana to Bitilasana (Cat/Cow Pose) with Variations

Come to your hands and knees, with your shoulders over your wrists and your knees at least hip-width apart. Inhale and gently arch your back, turning your gaze up toward the ceiling. Exhale as you round your back. Repeat this movement 5 times, with your eyes closed, visualizing your baby resting safely in the hammock of your belly.

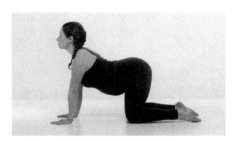 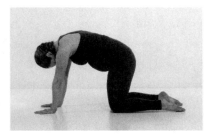

Pelvic Circles

Remain on your hands and knees, and begin to circle your hips, using the movements to explore your body and give your baby a little ride. Start with small circles, coordinating the movement with your breath, and then make them larger, if that feels comfortable.

BENEFITS: The combination of Marjaryasana and Bitilasana (Cat/Cow Pose) and Pelvic Circles alleviates back pain and stiffness as well as any pain you may be experiencing in your hip flexors.

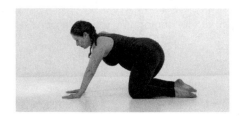 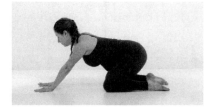

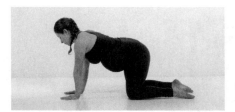 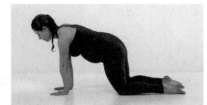

Thread the Needle

Come back to your hands and knees. Slightly engage your abdominal muscles to hug your baby gently as you reach your right arm out to the side and then thread it along the floor under your bent left arm until your right shoulder is on the floor. Rest your head on the floor or a block. Remain here for 3 breaths or more. Slowly press back up to your hands and knees and repeat on the other side.

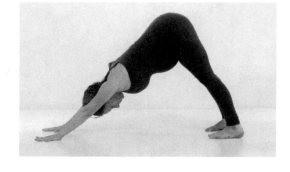

BENEFITS: This is a loving way to open space around your kidneys, upper back, and shoulders.

NOTE: Take the next few moments to string the last three poses together (Marjaryasana, Pelvic Circles, and Thread the Needle) in a sequence that feels like a natural flow or a gentle dance.

Adho Mukha Svanasana
(Downward-Facing Dog Pose)

Come into Adho Mukha Svanasana, placing your feet wider than your shoulders. Be still for a few breaths and simply experience the pose. From that place of deep listening, make any movements that will help you feel clearer in your body. Perhaps bend one leg, then the other, or both at the same time; rise onto the balls of your feet; or do Pelvic Circles with bent knees. Now commit to the pose by pressing your hands down and forward, while pulling your pelvis up and back to emphasize the length in your spine. Remain here for 3 breaths, as long as you feel comfortable.

BENEFITS: This pose stretches your back, shoulders, hips, and legs. It also lengthens your spine to give your baby more room and relieve any pressure on your uterus.

MODIFICATIONS: If at any time in your practice Adho Mukha Svanasana does not feel good, move into a nice, stretchy Uttana Shishosana (Extended Puppy Pose) instead.

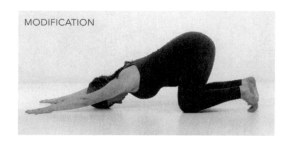

MODIFICATION

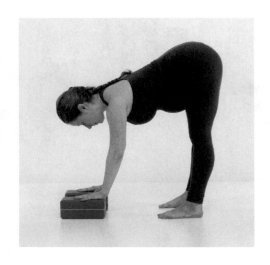

Uttanasana (Standing Forward Bend)

Bend your knees deeply and walk your feet toward your hands to come into Uttanasana with your back extended and your legs spaced wider than your hips. Place your hands on blocks that are far enough in front of you that your belly feels spacious and comfortable. Remain here for a few breaths, bend your knees, place your hands on your thighs one at a time, and slowly roll up to standing.

BENEFITS: This pose improves circulation in your legs, releases any tension in your neck and shoulders, and brings a sense of calm to your whole body.

Tadasana (Mountain Pose)

Stand with your feet wider than hip-width apart, which may be even a little wider than yesterday. For each foot, root the ball of your big toe, the ball of your little toe, and the center of your heel. Lift the arches of your feet, and from there, pull up the musculature of your legs. From the strong rooting of your base, let more space come between the discs of your spine.

BENEFITS: This pose improves your posture and helps correct any misalignments in your back and pelvic floor. Emotionally, it helps you feel confident and strong.

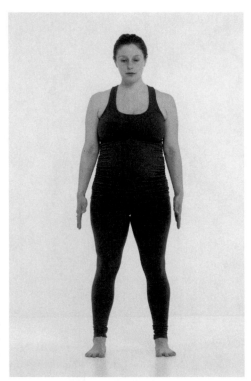

Pelvic Figure Eights

Standing in Tadasana (Mountain Pose), bend your knees slightly, and make slow figure eights with your pelvis. To do this, bring your right hip forward, then outward and around toward the right rear side. Then, on the diagonal, bring your left hip forward, circling around to the left rear side. Cut back diagonally to the front right. Repeat this motion as many times as you like, making it your own dance. Don't worry about doing it correctly; instead feel your hips, pelvis, uterus, and baby swirling around.

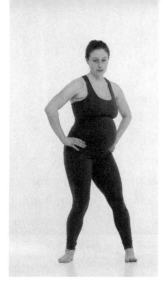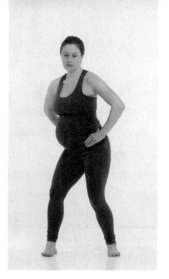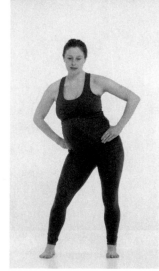

BENEFITS: This pose gives your baby a little ride while liberating your pelvic floor muscles. It provides a juicy experience for your hips, lower back, and pelvis, bringing fresh oxygenated blood and lymph to your pelvic region.

Surya Namaskar (Prenatal Sun Salutation)

Although these instructions are written with continuous movement and breath in mind, please feel free to take cues from your body and slow down and linger at any pose. Keep listening, and remember that you are your primary teacher.

Begin in Tadasana (Mountain Pose), with your feet at least hip-width apart. Inhale your arms up into Urdhva Hastasana (Upward Salute). As you exhale, take hold of your left wrist, lengthen on an inhalation, and exhale as you bend to your right. Inhale back to center, switch wrists, lengthen, and exhale as you bend to your left. Inhale back to center.

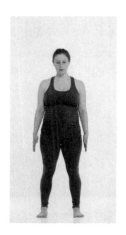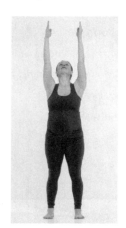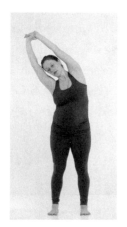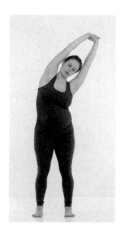

Exhale into Uttanasana (Standing Forward Bend), bending your knees enough to place your elbows on your thighs; press your palms together in prayer position at your heart. Remain here for a couple of breaths, expanding and releasing your pelvic floor; draw your pubic bone toward your tailbone and your sitting bones toward each other to engage your pelvic floor. Inhale up to Ardha Uttanasana (Half Standing Forward Bend) with your hands on blocks on the inside of your feet and your chest lifting forward. Exhale your right foot back into a high lunge and stay there for a few breaths, making sure your left knee is over your left ankle. Now place your hands on the ground. On your next exhalation, move into Adho Muhka Svanasana (Downward-Facing Dog Pose). Spend a few breaths visiting with dog pose, bending your knees as you see fit. Wrap your belly muscles around your baby, and inhale as you come forward into Phalakasana (Plank Pose) with very stable legs. Exhale as you lower your knees to the floor; walk your hands all the way back behind you for a modified Ustrasana (Camel Pose). Open your chest and lift your pelvis forward and up. Inhale to stay in the pose, then exhale as you lower your pelvis back down and walk your arms forward, back into Adho Mukha Svanasana.

Exhale your right foot forward to the outside of your right hand, or come down on your hands and knees and use your hand to draw your foot forward before raising your back knee up. Pause in a high lunge, then exhale and lower your left knee to the floor in Anjaneyasana (Low Lunge). Draw your right heel and your left knee toward each other to create stability and lift your arms to the sky. Bring your hands back down to the blocks, and straighten your left leg enough to push off and step forward to the outside of your left hand. Bend your knees, and return to bent-kneed Uttanasana, dropping heavily into your tailbone and heels. Roll up to Tadasana and breathe here for a few breaths.

For the next sequence, move to a wall.

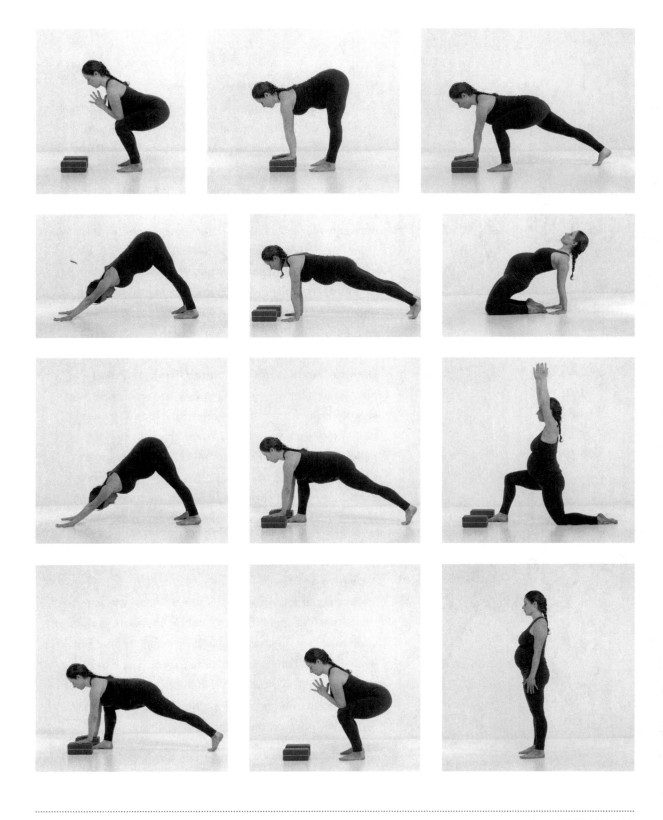

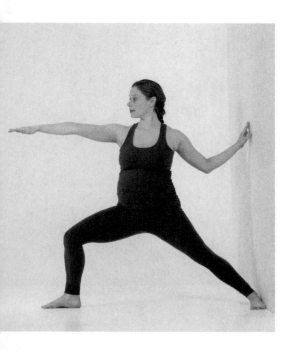

Virabhadrasana II (Warrior II Pose)

Take a wide stance with the outer edge of your left foot against a wall for balance and grounding. Now turn your right foot so it is perpendicular with the wall for Virabhadrasana II. Spread your toes and root through the four corners of each foot; bend your right knee and extend your arms out to the sides. As you feel the dynamic tension between your legs, breathe freedom into the length of your spine. Stay here, breathing normally, for 3 to 5 breaths or as long as you're comfortable. Repeat on the other side.

BENEFITS: This pose increases strength, flexibility, balance, and determination while energizing your whole body.

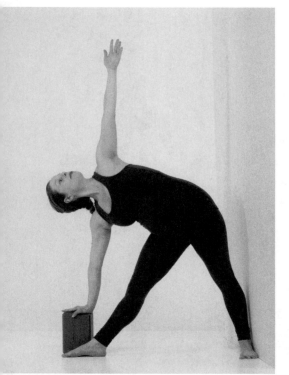

Utthita Trikonasana (Extended Triangle Pose)

Place your left heel against the wall and point your toes slightly away from it. Have your right foot and knee pointing directly forward. As in Virabhadrasana II (Warrior II Pose), start by finding your connection to the ground and let it rebound up through the crown of your head. Encourage active, strong legs. Reach your arms to the side, lean to your right, tipping your pelvis and baby over into Trikonasana. Place your hand on a block for an additional lift to ensure that your belly has enough room to feel expansive and free.

From your rooted left heel, turn your belly toward the sky as much as you feel comfortable, and expand through your arms. Soften your face, and be aware of your breath, even if it feels compromised because your baby has taken up some of your lung space. Stay in the pose for 2 to 3 breaths, or as long as you feel comfortable. Return to standing and repeat the pose on the other side.

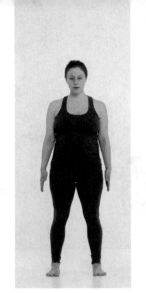
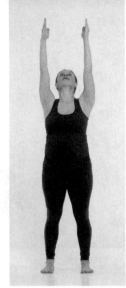

Tadasana (Mountain Pose) with Sound

Standing in Tadasana, inhale as you bring your arms up, and exhale as you bring them down. Allow your breath to be deep and long, and add low, sonorous sounds on every exhalation to open and release your pelvic floor.

BENEFITS: Low, deep sounds may encourage apana vayu and the downward movement of your baby into the birth canal.

Ardha Chandrasana (Half-Moon Pose)

With your whole back supported by a wall, step your feet out wide with your right foot pointing forward and the outside of your left foot against the wall. Holding a block with your right hand, bend your right knee and place the block several inches in front of your right foot, with your hand pressing down onto the block. Lift your left leg so it is roughly parallel to the floor and flex your foot. Allow the whole back of your body and head to lean against the wall. Remain here for several breaths, as long as you are comfortable. To come out of the pose, bend your right knee and carefully step your left foot down onto the mat. Repeat on the other side.

BENEFITS: Another powerful strengthening pose, Supported Ardha Chandrasana also engages your abdominals without gripping or putting pressure on your uterus.

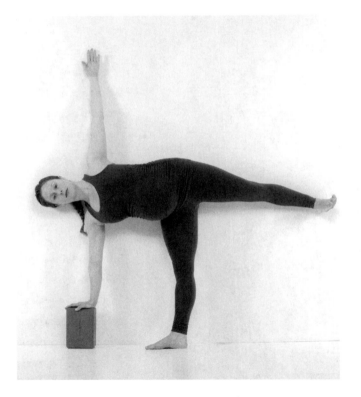

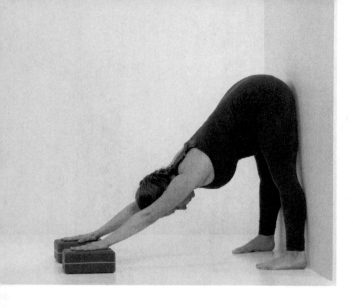

Prasarita Padottanasana (Wide-Legged Standing Forward Bend)

Still standing with your back at the wall, keep your stance wide. Bend forward from your hip joints, extending out through the crown of your head, and support your buttocks against the wall. Place your hands on blocks that are 3 to 4 feet in front of you. Keep your belly open, your spine long, and your shoulders relaxed. Stay here for several breaths, as long as you're comfortable.

BENEFITS: This pose improves circulation in your legs, releases your pelvic floor muscles, and relaxes your whole body.

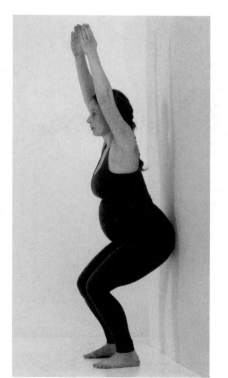

Utkatasana (Chair Pose)

From the preceding forward bend, heel-toe your feet in until they're slightly wider than hip-width. Press your sitting bones into the wall, lift your arms, and come into Utkatasana. Hold this pose for a full minute, if possible.

BENEFITS: A 1-minute hold is excellent preparation for labor, since 1 minute is the length of the average contraction.

Sacrum Massage

With your back still against the wall, bend your knees slightly, and use the wall to massage your sacrum. Move in circles, up and down, and back and forth, letting your intuition guide the tempo and pressure.

BENEFITS: A good release for your sacrum and lower back, this massage may also be useful during labor if your support team has gone on a break.

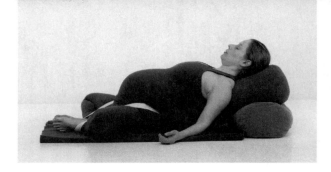

Supta Baddha Konasana
(Reclining Bound Angle Pose)

Place two bolsters behind you to form a T, with
the vertical bolster on top. Sit in front of the
bolsters with your bottom on the floor, your
knees bent, and your sacrum touching or slightly away from the bolster's
edge. Thread a strap from your sacrum around to the front of your thighs
and under your feet. Secure it loosely and tighten it after you lie back.
Place the soles of your feet together and open your knees. Now lie back
on the bolsters so your head and torso are supported and your legs and
buttocks are resting on the floor. Rest here for as long as you like.

MODIFICATION: During the last month or two of pregnancy, place a block
between your feet to broaden your pelvis and release the pelvic floor muscles.

BENEFITS: This pose creates more room in your pelvis and releases any
gripping in your pelvic floor muscles. The gentle backbend also opens your
shoulders and releases tension in your neck and upper back.

Side-Lying Savasana (Corpse Pose)

Lying on your left side, straighten your left leg. Bend your right leg and place
the knee, shin, and foot on a bolster that you've positioned in front of and
parallel to your straight left leg. (Don't put the bolster between your legs; only
under the top, bent knee.) Rest your head on a folded blanket so that it's in
line with your spine and, if you wish, place your top arm on a folded blanket
or bolster. Remain in the pose for as long as you like, at least 3 to 5 minutes.

BENEFIT: A deeply relaxing pose to soothe your nervous system, soften
any rough emotional edges, and relieve fatigue. Almost as good as sleeping,
which can sometimes be elusive.

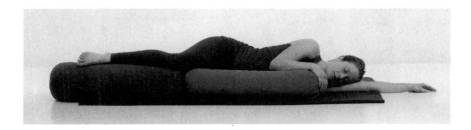

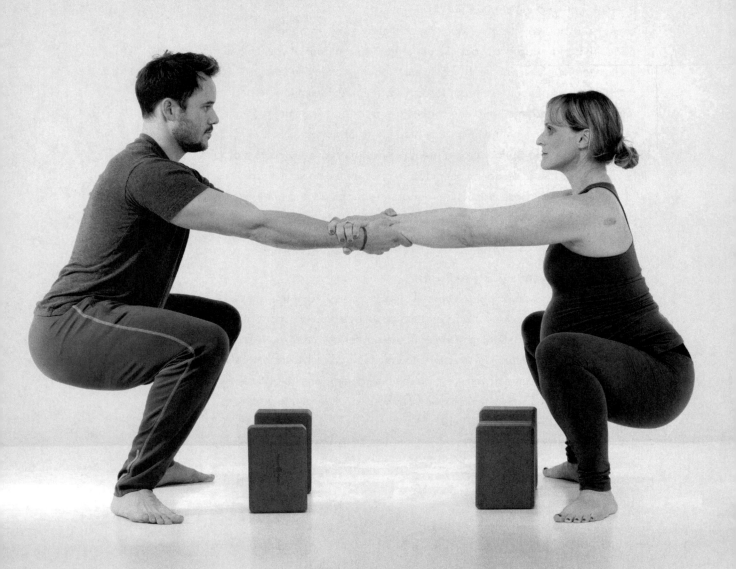

5.

LABOR AND BIRTHING

Connection and Support
From Thirty-Seven to Forty-Two Weeks

Sequences by De West

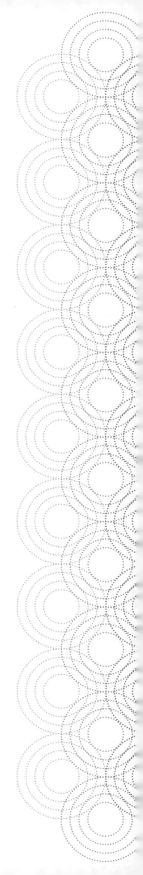

All of the yoga, pranayama, reading, and deep listening you've done and all the conversations you've had over the past nine months (give or take a few weeks) have prepared you for this moment. Your labor is about to begin, and you will soon be holding your baby in your arms. Of course, *soon* is a relative term, but clearly you've entered the home stretch. In the next few days or in a couple of weeks, you will transition from being pregnant to giving birth, as your baby continues to drop into place and your cervix widens to accommodate her descent. You may be feeling impatient by now. After all, there are only so many times you can fold and refold baby clothes, rearrange the nursery, or bemoan the fact that your confident stride has turned into a duck-like waddle. Or perhaps you have an overwhelming urge to create something—draw, paint, sculpt, bake, or write—or conversely, to retreat and reflect. Don't be surprised if you dissolve into a giant puddle of tears one minute and a jumble of anxious thoughts the next, only to feel giddy with excitement soon after that.

Instead of feeling stuck or frustrated that your pregnancy will never end, think of this time as a prelude to what's coming. The definition of *prelude* ("the introduction to something more important") implies expectation, a sense of excitement, like a prelude to a kiss or an opening to a grand piece of orchestral music. It's a time of mindful, even eager anticipation in which you watch, wait, and move to the rhythm of your own experience. You get to adapt everything, including your yoga practice, to honor whatever your body and your mind need right now. Indeed, as uncomfortable as you may feel, this time is precious. Whether you're pregnant with your first child or you've been through this scenario before, saying good-bye to the old you and opening physically and emotionally to your new life can be both exhilarating and a bit daunting. As yoga has taught you so often, though, returning to the power of the breath can be your ally as your practice shifts to accommodate the physical changes you're experiencing, the emotional roller coaster you may be riding, and the journey your baby is about to take.

A few years ago, Jana Studelska, a licensed midwife who practices in northern Minnesota and Wisconsin, wrote an article in *Mothering* magazine, in which she called these last few days of pregnancy a *zwischen* (German for "between"), "where mothers linger, waiting to be called forward." Naming this time, she says, "gives it dimension, an experience closer to wonder than endurance." Doing slow-moving poses at this point in your journey can bring you to a place of deep self-inquiry, in which you can simultaneously surrender and embrace. You may be able to begin to let go of any muscular or emotional resistance you have to giving birth and simply sit with what is, even if what is doesn't feel that great or is fraught with anxiety, sadness, fear, or impatience. During this "closer to wonder" time, perhaps you will discover and begin to trust your strength and your instinctive ability to mother your newborn child.

Don't skimp on zwischen or your commitment to practice during that time. Staying present as your third trimester comes to a close and you move into the more active stages of labor can prepare you mentally and emotionally for the intensity of the work ahead of you. Practicing yoga (on both a physical and philosophical level) can help you approach labor and birthing more with reverence and surrender than fear and uncertainty. But before exploring how to do that, a look at what's going on in your body is in order.

The Inside Scoop

Throughout your pregnancy your endocrine system has produced hormones such as hCG, estrogen, progesterone, and relaxin that expand, contain, and nurture your body. These hormones have allowed your ligaments and muscles to soften to accommodate your growing uterus, while simultaneously making sure nothing gets rejected or leaves too soon; they've begun to prime your breasts for milk production and they've increased your body's blood and fluid levels substantially to deliver nutrients to your baby.

A slightly different collection of hormones must now orchestrate your baby's birth by stimulating your body to squeeze, expel, envelop, and welcome. Basically four types of hormones take center stage now: oxytocin, beta-endorphins, adrenaline/noradrenaline, and prolactin—all of which are stress hormones. The complex interplay of these hormones originates deep within the primitive brain and is not fully understood. But we do know that oxytocin causes contractions and a sense of connection; beta-endorphins lessen pain and often bring the mother into an altered state of consciousness; adrenaline and noradrenaline, the fight-or-flight hormones, either slow down or speed up labor, depending on what's needed; and prolactin, the mothering or nesting hormone, gets the milk flowing.

SQUEEZE AND EXPEL

Oxytocin, manufactured in the hypothalamus and distributed in pulses from the pituitary gland, controls the frequency and intensity of contractions that dilate and thin the cervix, giving the baby room to enter and move through the birth canal. In an uninterrupted birth, oxytocin increases near the end of labor and in concert with the other hormones creates a burst of strong contractions that help push the baby out quickly and easily. It also helps eject the placenta, prevent hemorrhaging, and stimulate the milk letdown reflex so a mother can breastfeed her baby.

Beta-endorphins act as the body's natural pain relievers, often giving the mother an "other worldly" sense of transcending the pain. They work particularly well when she feels warm, safe, and loved; in other words, when oxytocin levels are high. Sarah Buckley, MD, a New Zealand–trained physician and the author of *Gentle Birth, Gentle Mothering* points out that very high levels of beta-endorphins will reduce oxytocin levels and slow down labor, "which may help to ration the intensity according to our ability to deal with it."

Adrenaline and noradrenaline protect the mother and baby from harm. If the mother senses danger or is interrupted in any way during labor, these fight-or-flight hormones kick in to slow contractions way down until the perceived threat has diminished. At the end of labor, they'll again pick up the pace so that the mother has the strength and energy to push her baby out.

ENVELOP AND WELCOME

Oxytocin, the love or cuddle hormone, also plays a role in feelings of well-being and connection and even the ability to trust. Babies produce oxytocin too, according to Dr. Buckley, so in the moments right after birth, "both mother and baby are bathed in this ecstatic cocktail of hormones," which is increased by skin-to-skin and eye-to-eye contact and by the baby attaching to the mother's breast. Beta-endorphins join with oxytocin to increase a sense of post-labor bliss and even help the body release prolactin, the mothering hormone that gets the milk flowing. Prolactin also triggers an emotional and behavioral response that helps mothers put their babies' needs first. Combined with oxytocin right after birth, Dr. Buckley says prolactin "encourages a relaxed and selfless devotion to the baby that contributes to a mother's satisfaction and her baby's physical and emotional health." The levels of fight-or-flight hormones plummet after a woman gives birth so that oxytocin can continue to increase to keep mother and baby connected in a loving way (and to prevent postpartum bleeding).

Sadly, all of this exquisite interplay among the birthing hormones doesn't happen as seamlessly or as strongly when the labor and birth need medical assistance. Dr. Buckley points out that peak levels of oxytocin at the end of labor can't occur when a woman has received an epidural, and not achieving those levels can interfere with the bonding between mother and baby. Synthetic oxytocin (such as Pitocin, for example), which mothers are sometimes given to jump-start stalled labor, does not contribute to the post-birth high like naturally occurring oxytocin, and can actually interfere with the mother's own oxytocin system, she says. Synthetic oxytocin can start contractions before the body's natural opiates, the beta-endorphins, are activated to lessen the pain. As a consequence, those labor pains are generally intense but not always as effective. So our best chance at a natural childbirth occurs when there's as little interference—medically, socially, and even personally—as possible.

MINIMIZING INTERRUPTIONS

Because the intricate dance of hormones necessary to birth your baby happens in the deepest part of your brain (the primitive limbic system, or what scientists call the mammalian brain)—a place beyond your conscious control—thinking too much interrupts the process. Dr. Buckley says that the act of giving birth "is exquisitely sensitive to outside influences, and anything that disturbs a laboring woman's sense of safety and privacy will disrupt [it]." According to Dr. Buckley, bright lights, fetal monitoring, moving from one place to another, conversation, and even expectations from your more rational mind (the neocortex) can often prolong labor and make things more difficult. In fact, the more we intervene in the process, the more awry our birthing hormones can go, and the more problems we are likely to create. The bottom line: When a woman feels safe, has enough privacy, and isn't "on display," she can more easily surrender control, allowing the natural birthing process to proceed. As a body-based meditation practice, yoga prepares us to do that, to trust the body's innate wisdom—a necessary practice for childbirth—without trying to steer it in a particular direction. When we give birth, we also must shed our ego and get out of the way of the process. Sometimes that dissolution of ego is an ecstatic one, as Dr. Buckley reminds us, and sometimes the process is painful.

Visualizing what will happen during your labor may help you flow with the process a little more easily and not resist or feel frightened. In fact, Ina May Gaskin, the near-legendary midwife, cofounder of The Farm Midwifery Center in Tennessee, and the author of several books on natural childbirth, says, "We need to always remember that mothers who are afraid tend to secrete the hormones that delay or inhibit birth. This is true of all mammals and is part of nature's design. Those who are not terrified are more likely to secrete in abundance the hormones that make labor and birth easier and less painful—sometimes even pleasurable."

Think of the uterus as a giant upside-down pear, with the cervix at the smallest end of the fruit. The three layers of strong yet flexible muscle fiber that line the uterine walls expand as the baby grows; in fact, by the time you go into labor, the top of the uterus is pressing up against your lower ribcage. The middle layer of the uterus, the myometrium, contains the smooth muscle, which is what contracts and shortens during labor. The cervix is a band of strong muscles that has steadfastly held the contents of the uterus safe and must now get thin enough (efface) to open (dilate) wide enough for the baby to come through the expanded vaginal opening. To help visualize effacement, imagine your baby's head pushing through a turtleneck sweater.

THE NEED FOR PRIVACY

I began to understand the need for privacy and safety when Dr. Buckley explained that the act of giving birth was a lot like making love—even the same hormones are at play. Could you imagine making love with people coming in and out of the room, interrupting you, asking questions, turning on the lights, and monitoring your blood pressure to see if you're about to climax? "The parallels between making love and giving birth became very clear to me," Dr. Buckley says, "not only in terms of passion and love, but also because we need essentially the same conditions for both experiences: to feel private, safe, and unobserved." Several studies back her up, suggesting that when women have privacy and feel safe, they have an easier time (shorter births, fewer interventions) than when they are subjected to outside influences.

We're really not so different from animals in the wild who instinctively leave their pack, flock, or herd and find a private space when they're ready to give birth. Or even from our pets who choose a laundry basket or the back of a closet. If anything interrupts them, their fight-or-flight response will slow down their labor and, until danger passes, actually prevent birth from taking place. The same thing can happen to us. Anything that makes a woman anxious, distracted, or confused—that is, anything that takes her from an internal focus to an external one—can cause stress and alter her ability to give birth. Many women find that their labor will slow down, for example, when they go from home to hospital. Some even report going from five or six centimeters dilated back to three centimeters when people they've never met begin asking personal questions, the lights are bright, the room is sterile, and they're given a hospital gown to put on as though they were ill.

Making Friends with Pain

Before we explore the stages of labor, let's address the elephant in the room: pain. How much will all this hurt? Most women admit that the pain of childbirth is right up at the top of their worry list, often before they even get pregnant, and their fear only intensifies as their due date approaches. They hear horror stories from friends, read far too many accounts of 40-hour labors that ended in cesarean births, and even get advice from well-meaning doctors to schedule an epidural ahead of time to mitigate the pain that will surely be too much to handle.

No one likes to be in pain. Pain generally signals that something is wrong and we need to fix it. No wonder many women automatically request pain medication even before their labor starts. In fact, when my daughter Megan took a tour of the birthing center near her home, the other women in the group couldn't believe she wanted a natural childbirth. All they wanted to know was whether they could still get pain meds if they chose the birthing center and how quickly they could get them. A couple of women even wondered if they should simply schedule a cesarean birth so they wouldn't feel a thing.

Sadly, these women aren't an anomaly. Elective epidural use has risen over the years and now, according to the Centers for Disease Control and Prevention, at least 60 percent (some statistics say 70 percent) of women use some kind of anesthesia when giving birth.

The Sphincter Law

Ina May Gaskin says a failure to respect what she's coined the Sphincter Law is probably responsible for most obstetrical interventions and a woman's difficulty in letting go of the pelvic floor. Basically, sphincters are groups of muscles that tighten around bodily orifices—such as the anus, cervix, and vagina—to keep them closed, and then relax when they need to open. Sphincters function best when you have privacy. You can't have a bowel movement, for example, when someone is watching you to make sure you do it right; the same holds true for making love and giving birth. The sphincters won't open on command, Gaskin says, and if you "become upset, frightened, humiliated, or self-conscious," high levels of stress hormones like adrenaline and cortisol may cause them to shut down.

I would never suggest that a woman who asked for an epidural or had to have a cesarean birth (especially on the advice of her midwife or doula) made the wrong decision or chose a harmful path. What's most important is that we follow our own knowing in order to birth our babies. No matter what your birthing experience is like, you will probably look back on it as one of the most challenging, powerful, and awe-inspiring moments in your life.

Fortunately, your yoga practice may help you approach labor in a way that can allow you to welcome the pain instead of pushing it away or feeling victimized by it. In fact, if you've been doing yoga for a while, you've probably already experienced two types of pain: a searing, stabbing pain that grips your back, knee, ankle, or shoulder when you've either gone too far in a pose, fallen out of one, or aggravated an old injury; and an aching, sometimes shaky, discomfort when you've held a pose for longer than you're used to and your muscles begin to stretch uncomfortably as they open and then release. Just the language we use for those two types of pain is instructive: we grip and tighten against destructive pain, trying to figure out how to get it to stop and what kind of damage it signals; we open and release when the pain is constructive, welcoming it even as we stay engaged with the sensation.

Practicing svadhyaya, you can begin to listen a little deeper: What is this pain telling you? How do you access it, and from that place, how can you begin to release the gripping muscles and soften around the discomfort? Instead of resisting the pain, can you invite it in? Just like on your yoga mat, if you can remember that the pain you experience in childbirth is born of expansion and release—a signal that everything is working as it should—you may be able move through it, knowing that it's helping your baby into the birth canal.

Stephanie Snyder, the San Francisco yoga teacher who created the second trimester sequence in Chapter 2, said she really couldn't wrap her head around the pain during her first birthing experience. When she looked back on her first labor, she told me, she realized that she was resisting the contractions "because they were, well, *uncomfortable*." That resistance caused her to back away from the pain, to try and get around it somehow. Practicing prenatal yoga during her second pregnancy helped her figure out how to "soften into the discomfort." She consciously chose to trust that her body and her baby knew exactly what to do and when to do it. When she realized that every contraction was helping her baby move down and out, she welcomed the sensation, letting go of "me" and collaborating instead of resisting.

As always, look to your breath to gauge your level of anxiety and resistance and to help you calm down and focus. It's easy for women to lose control of their breath, either holding it or constricting it, when they fixate on the pain. When that happened to my friend Janice, her husband Will put on a chanting playlist and she began to chant. Her attention and energy, which felt lodged in her chest, quickly began to move downward, back into her pelvis. When her voice grew hoarse, Will chanted for her. Just like on your mat, you can inhale to expand your capacity, find a little more space around a sensation, and then exhale your attention deeper into your experience, releasing any muscular or emotional resistance.

Support in Many Guises

As many female yoga practitioners have discovered, you can't do everything by yourself. We learn on our mats that there are times to stand on our own two feet, discovering where our strengths and challenges lie, and times to reach out for support. That support can present itself as inanimate objects—straps, bolsters, blankets, and blocks—or as loving encouragement and assistance from a teacher or another student in class. Although no one knows your body as intimately as you do, your yoga teacher can encourage you to try new things, such as showing you ways to open more fully in a backbend without compromising your lower back or exploring poses you thought weren't available to you in a safe and appropriate way. The language of support used on the yoga mat and in a yoga practice is the same language you need to conjure for labor and birthing. Just like a good teacher, a good coach in labor and birthing is invaluable. Studies abound to show that medical interventions decrease considerably when a woman enlists the help of a midwife or a doula.

Real Facts about Medical Interventions

Although I had made the commitment to a natural childbirth, I had no idea what would happen or even if I could handle the pain of it all. Luckily, a nurse practitioner/midwife sat me down and explained all the reasons why I should think twice before I called for medication:

- An epidural would actually slow down (read: prolong) my labor, and why would I want to do that?
- An epidural would prevent me from walking or even changing positions often during labor. I wanted gravity to assist me; being confined to a bed, on my back, hooked up to monitors and IVs feels counterproductive.
- Research shows that epidurals can increase both the possibility of needing to have a vacuum- or forceps-assisted birth and the likelihood of having a cesarean birth.
- Since an epidural slows down labor, its use may increase the need for labor-inducing medications like Pitocin to jump-start the body's natural process again. Pitocin actually makes labor pains more intense, but alas, not necessarily more effective.
- An epidural interrupts the delicate balance of hormonal activity necessary for an optimal birthing experience for mother and baby. I wanted to trust my body's natural abilities.
- An epidural would interfere with my ability to bond with my baby after her birth and might increase postpartum pains, making recovery more difficult.

In addition to all that, I'm more afraid of the side effects of medications than I am of pain. So when I heard that epidurals can sometimes cause headaches, backaches, nausea, a drop in blood pressure, and a spike in body temperature, I made a conscious effort to avoid them, if at all possible.

Even with this type of assistance, sometimes the support you need isn't what you envisioned in the first place: medication to jumpstart your labor or an epidural to stop the pain. Because of the side effects and risks involved, I would caution you to make intervention decisions like these in concert with your birthing team and your own body's needs, not just on the advice of your OB/GYN. At certain times, appropriate use of medication is very helpful. Some women, for example, can't seem to let go of the grip on their pelvic muscles, so they need help releasing those muscles and creating more space in their pelvic floor for the baby to exit; other times, they may need a respite if their labor has dragged on for hours. In researching this topic, I was happy to learn that doctors can give just enough pain support to give mamas a break but still allow them to push their babies out effectively. My friend Einav Keet, a writer from Philadelphia, told me that she endured thirty-six hours of not-very-productive labor, until her doctor encouraged her to get an epidural so she could rest and have the energy to push. "I was exhausted and realized I'd hit an energy wall," she says. "Luckily, the epidural wore off in time for me to push, which felt amazing."

NOTE: If you do decide on an epidural and are instructed not to move around, you can still use your yoga breathing techniques to birth your baby effectively. Ask your midwife or doctor to help you to move to a side-lying position with your top leg slightly elevated instead of remaining flat on your back.

Moving through the Stages

When women think about going into labor they often divide that journey into two parts: early labor where the pain is pretty manageable, and active labor (first and second stage) where it becomes increasingly intense and sometimes unbearable. They tend to dismiss the in-between time as nothing special, just a waiting game punctuated by the commonly uttered sentiments, *I can't wait to have this baby!* and *I am so sick of being pregnant!* And they get frustrated by the starts and stops of what obstetricians call false labor and midwives call embarkment. These two stages are important, however, because they can set the pace for the entire experience by giving women the opportunity to go slow and stay in close contact with their inner knowing. By the time they move into labor in earnest, they feel more prepared and more able to participate fully in the process.

A TIME IN BETWEEN

I like to think of zwischen as a dress rehearsal, a necessary preamble to labor and birthing, during which a mama's heart begins to open (along with her cervix). To give birth, midwife Jana Studelska says a woman must realize that "every resource she has will be called on to assist in this journey," and spending this time calling forth these resources will make her feel more prepared. This statement is akin to what your yoga practice asks of you on a daily basis: stay rooted in the physical sensations of your experience and listen to your body's cues. So many of us get into trouble when we allow our minds to dictate what the body should and shouldn't do, when we extend beyond our capacity. Mr. Iyengar says we extend from the intellect or the mind, but we expand our awareness from the heart. You have entered into heart time! You have everything you need to give birth to your baby. You have the same physical strength and mental resolve as countless women who came before you, as well as a heartful willingness, born of diligent practice, to dive deep inside your experience—in all its messiness—without judgment. Your ability to set aside things that don't ring true for you will help you resist outside pressure to make decisions that don't feel right and, at the same time, be okay with whatever birthing experience you end up having.

No matter what you're experiencing right now, give yourself permission to do whatever feels good at the moment: stretch, sing, chant, walk, make love, wail, cry, laugh, sleep. The ayurvedic specialist Niika Quistgard counsels her prenatal clients to practice the yoga of sound: sing, chant, or tone. The power of your voice, she says, "can awaken and amplify your innate strength, your faith in your body, and your trust in the goodness of life." Singing, chanting, or toning can be a sweet practice as you prepare to birth your baby. And of course, your baby will love hearing you croon.

Don't worry if you're not much of a singer—your baby certainly won't mind. Niika suggests toning instead; it's a simple technique that you may find effective all through zwischen and during labor, either by itself or in conjunction with slow mini vinyasa sequences, such as the Mama Salutes on page 168 that De West offers. In toning, you sustain one long vowel sound on a single note, which Niika says supports a relaxed focus and breath control during labor, and it may help you meet and ride the contractions that move through your system. Toning is easy to practice. Simply sit in a comfortable position, with your hands on your belly. Inhale fully, and as you exhale, maintain a long "ooh" or "aah" sound until your breath is finished. Then inhale and tone again. Do this as many times as you wish, allowing yourself to feel the power of the vibration moving through your whole being. You may end up toning a sound that's more a mixture of a chant and a moan, but the vibration of whatever sound you make will calm your nervous system and soothe your baby.

Whenever the opportunity arises or the spirit moves you, get up and dance around your living room. Niika calls dancing the best way to "invite your nervous system to feel the joy of simply being," which can take a little of the seriousness out of "laboring." Plus, it's a fun way to connect movement with breath and encourage your baby to move into place. Dancing is almost always guaranteed to make you feel beautiful and confident and, as Niika puts it, ready "to open completely to all that unfolds along this incredible transformative journey."

EMBARKMENT

At some point during this in-between time, you'll probably begin to experience contractions. Your doctor may very well tell you that what you feel is nothing more than "false labor," and that true labor doesn't start until your contractions have found their rhythm and are coming at regular intervals. There's really nothing false about your labor. Childbirth educator Jane Austin prefers to call it the warm-up. You might not feel like much is happening, but this is actually a rich stage, one that can last just a few hours or as long as a week or more. Psychologically, you've started to move from your rational, thinking mind into your more embodied, intuitive mind in order to open the lines of communication even wider between you and your baby. Your baby is busy, too, as Ina May Gaskin puts it in her *Guide to Childbirth*, being "pushed, jostled, wriggled, and turned into the most advantageous position" for birth.

Physiologically, the cervix has definitely begun to efface and become softer, and the mucus plug that seals off the cervix may pass, leaving behind a brownish or pinkish, mucusy discharge. The cervix may also start to dilate a little, especially if the baby's head is sitting directly on it.

Some women feel intense, intermittent contractions during embarkment; others may experience cramping, almost like menstrual discomfort; while still others may feel nothing at all. But regardless of what you feel or don't feel, things are definitely happening. You may also be experiencing some Braxton-Hicks gripping, those silent, belly-tightening sensations you've probably had for a number of months. Not true contractions per se, they work to condition and tone the uterus in preparation for labor. Embarkment, on the other hand, consists of coordinated contractions that thin and open the cervix and move the baby along.

Calling this time "false labor" can be counterproductive. In yoga we are taught that our language—how we talk about and communicate with our bodies—has a huge impact on how we think about and interact with ourselves. "False labor" makes it sound like your body has done something to fool or betray you, purposely setting up a situation to prove you can't trust it. Not a great way to go into labor together. Thinking of this time as a warm-up instead will give you an opportunity to ease into your experience, a little like the warm-up you do in yoga class before you begin the more intense part of the sequence—centering your energy as you bring your attention into the room, waking up your body and connecting your breath with your movements. When you approach the earliest stage of labor in the same way, Jane Austin says, "You realize that your body is doing exactly what it needs to be doing. You understand what you need to do, and you can move into full-on labor from that place of being held and loved." These warm-up coordinated contractions often happen at night when you're asleep. Why? Quite possibly because your level of oxytocin (those contraction-producing hormones) is highest in an environment in which you feel safe, warm, and cared for.

Your Yoga Practice Take time now to practice yoga sequences that incorporate deep, low sound—from chanting and deep Ujjayi humming to full-out moaning—to encourage your baby to press down on your cervix to cause it to open. As you do these poses (the Flowing with the Breath sequence on page 166), remember to keep your jaw and face soft and relaxed, which in turn will soften and release your pelvis, and to direct the sound all the way to your pelvic floor. Use low guttural notes; their vibration will help to create a calm connection to the earth and reach deep into your pelvis.

Continue to practice conscious breathing techniques. Smooth, steady breaths can balance your nervous system, calm your mind, and allow your endocrine system (where the hormones come from) to function properly. Now is a good time to practice Samavrtti Pranayama (Even Breathing) (see page 155). Doing poses that will allow you to move around and change positions, employing a downward movement of apana vayu, can stimulate labor, and the pull of gravity will help your baby move down and into position.

As mentioned earlier, it's not always easy, but try feeling grateful for each letting go instead of tensing against the pain. Gurmukh gives us a powerful reminder: "Fear cannot live in thankfulness." Whenever you feel as though you can't do this, that it's just too much, come back to your breath and send a message of gratitude to your baby. Ina May Gaskin, one of my birthing heroes, expands on Gurmukh's teaching in a most yogic way: "With relief and gratitude comes a rush of endorphins, nature's opiates. Pain diminishes, [which] causes still more relief and gratitude and a stronger endorphin effect . . . When a mother starts to understand that being amused and grateful actually moves the process of labor along more efficiently, she starts to work toward these feelings herself. Hard work may continue, but she now has the heart for it. Instead of fearing her body, she experiments with trusting it."

EARLY LABOR

At some point, you'll start to notice that your labor pains have become more regular (eventually around five minutes apart), are getting stronger, and are lasting a bit longer (about forty-five seconds to a minute), as your cervix continues to ripen and pull back. For some women, early labor contractions are still manageable; for others, they can be fairly intense. Continue to do anything that feels good to you. You may want to keep walking, dancing, or doing gentle yoga, particularly poses that encourage you to move your hips and pelvis. Walking meditation not only allows gravity to assist the baby's descent (which opens your cervix more), but it can also help you stay focused on your internal sensations. Plus it gives you something to do so you don't feel anxious or impatient. Walking with your partner or midwife is nice because you'll have someone to lean on during contractions. Slow, fluid yoga moves, like those described in Chapter 3, can encourage your pelvic floor muscles to release and your bones to shift to give your baby more wiggle room. Do these asanas with your eyes closed so you can keep your attention in your body and connect your movements with your breath. Of course, getting some rest and eating when you're hungry are equally important in early labor. Both relaxing and eating will help you store up some energy you'll need when labor becomes more intense.

Although several studies suggest that women who labor and give birth in the comfort and privacy of their own homes often have an easier time, not every woman will want to do that or feel that she can. But with some planning and the support of a midwife or doula, you can still create a safe, inviting atmosphere within a hospital setting that will allow you to stay in your own rhythm and have the experience you envision. If you are planning a hospital birth, resist the urge to pack up and go there until the last possible moment. Your doula or midwife can help you make that decision. Instead, remain with those you love in a place that feels private and safe for as long as you can. Interacting with people you don't know in a sometimes chaotic, confusing atmosphere can slow your labor way down, which for some doctors signals the need for medical intervention.

Ban the Clocks

Although knowing what to expect helps many women go into labor consciously and without a lot of fear and anxiety, getting too hung up on the different stages and what they mean can actually slow things down. Jane Austin tells all her birthing mothers to get rid of or cover up any clock in their birthing room. Being so focused on what stage you're in or how many minutes have passed between contractions takes you out of your internal experience and engages your rational mind, which could easily prolong your labor. Instead, pay attention to what is actually happening to you, and don't be surprised when things happen and change quickly, then slow to a crawl again.

Jump-Start Stalled Labor

If your labor doesn't seem to be progressing, you can bump up the hormone volume without resorting to pharmaceuticals. Having sex is the best way. Oxytocin is responsible not only for contractions but also for orgasms—they don't call it the love hormone for nothing! Nipple stimulation also increases oxytocin. The rhythmic yoga, walking, and dancing you're doing may increase contractions or at least make them more efficient. So will taking a shower or relaxing in a warm tub. You can also ask your midwife or OB/GYN to strip the membranes, which means gently separating the amniotic sac from the cervix. Ina May Gaskin states that this method has been successful in a number of cases. Just make sure your doctor or midwife has experience in this procedure; you don't want your water to break yet.

ACTIVE LABOR—FIRST STAGE

After a while—and that "while" varies widely from woman to woman and birth to birth—your laboring sensations will come more frequently (every two or three minutes), last longer (at least a minute), and be more insistent. Your baby's head is pressing harder on your pelvic outlet, eager to make his way out. You may have trouble walking or interacting with anyone at this point. If that's the case, you should call your midwife or doula, if you haven't already. If you've chosen a hospital birth, you and your support team should probably go there now.

Regardless of where you decide to give birth, stay close to your experience. Use your exhalations to ride the contractions downward, visualize your baby's head moving through that snug turtleneck sweater, and rest whenever and however you can. Remember the definition of *yoga* is the union of opposites: within every effort, we can find ease; every contraction contains a release downward; every breath cycle includes a rest stop. Also remember that your body knows how much intensity you can bear—it has a built-in system for doling out contractions and providing natural opiates to soften the pain, giving space to rest between contractions, and even pulling back on contractions when they prove to be too much.

Sometimes the hardest things we have to do are to stay with it, not give up, and trust that the system won't fail us. Once again, humming, toning, or making any kind of sounds will help you stay connected with your breath.

Try to rest as fully as you can between contractions, calling on your yoga breathing to reenergize yourself for the next sensation. This in-between time can be an experience of profound stillness. Once active labor kicks in, if you have trouble finding the rhythm of your breath, ask your midwife or partner to do pranayama or chant, sing, or hum along with you. If you get lost, their steadiness can bring you back to the present.

Your Yoga Practice Do whatever feels good and whatever will persuade your pelvic floor to relax and open. Cat/Cow stretches on all fours will encourage your baby to roll his spine along your belly, which creates the easiest and least painful exit strategy. When you inhale and arch, make sure to engage your belly muscles a little bit (think of it as hugging your baby in) so you don't put too much pressure on your lower back. If arching hurts your back, keep your spine neutral. Gentle rocking from side to side on a big exercise ball may give you more support. The poses beginning on page 92 (Polar Bear Pose, Pelvic Circles, and Figure Eights) can be done on all fours or standing up and holding on to your partner for support. Try both the regular and the asymmetrical squats on pages 163–64, with your partner holding you under your armpits. "Spooning" with your partner in a sidesaddle Savasana does double duty: it helps you get the rest and support you need between contractions, and the extra cuddling increases your oxytocin levels to assist you in birthing your baby.

If your labor doesn't appear to be progressing, it could be because your baby's head isn't quite centered on your cervix. My daughter Megan's contractions, though mild, kept a pretty steady pace, increasing when she showered and walked but stalling out when she sat down. After a few hours of this, her doula noticed that the baby's head was off to the right, so while Megan was almost completely effaced, her cervix hadn't begun to dilate much. A combination of pelvic floor postures, a special side-lying pose from spinningbabies.com (see Resources), and Ina May Gaskin's famous "Shaking the Apples" routine (see below), jostled him into position. A warm bath, a little glass of wine, and a good night's sleep helped Megan calm her nerves, and she went into active labor in earnest early the next morning.

Shaking the Apples

Come onto all fours and move into Uttana Shoshosana (Puppy Pose) with your arms stretched out in front of you and your sitting bones lifting toward the ceiling. Have your partner or doula get behind you and jiggle your upper thighs vigorously one at a time (or both at once if a shawl or rebozo is used).

BENEFITS: This is good for loosening your pelvic floor muscles, anytime during labor, especially if your mind is too tense to let go. It works particularly well in conjunction with a "double hip squeeze" in which your partner or doula applies pressure to the outside of both hips, moving them toward the midline. You can see an example of the double hip squeeze in the partner sequence on page 164.

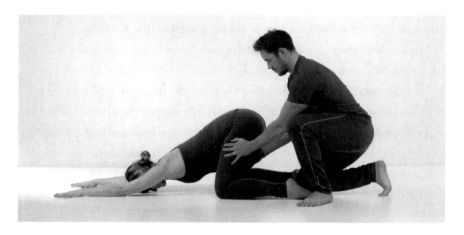

ACTIVE LABOR—SECOND STAGE

Generally speaking, this stage (which lasts from transition until birth) is the most intense, but it doesn't usually last as long as the first active stage, especially if you've had at least one baby already. The powerful sensations can be a little disorienting though, so you may have a difficult time figuring out what you need from moment to moment. Don't even try.

Keep your focus turned inward as much as you can. Ask for what you want, even if that's for people to leave. Don't think you have to be logical or even aware of other people's feelings. One moment you may want a gentle massage from your partner or midwife to relieve some of the intensity you're feeling. Two minutes later, you may not want to be disturbed at all—no talking, no music, no lights. And suddenly, you need to be in the tub. That's all perfect and perfectly in tune.

Gentle yoga movements, like Pelvic Circles, in a warm-water bath; chanting while slowly changing position (from squatting to all fours to lying on your side); moving with your baby's journey in mind—all of these are good strategies to keep your focus inward and your baby moving downward. Breathing techniques like Rose Petal Breath (see page 117) keep your attention on your breath, your lips and throat soft, and your cervix pliable and open.

Yoga helped me ride the intensity of transition and give birth to both of my daughters naturally, not solely because I used its breathing techniques and gravity-encouraging positions. Yoga taught me to ride the waves of sensation whenever I hold a difficult pose for several minutes. By doing so, I discovered that I could stay in discomfort for five minutes (or maybe five breaths) and not dissolve or expire. Of course, realizing that the whole process was almost over and that my baby just needed some extra-powerful contractions so she could make her debut also kept me going.

Your Yoga Practice

As most yoga practitioners know, yoga comes from the Sanskrit verb *yuj*, which means "to yoke or join together." Yoga is the way to unite the seemingly disparate parts of yourself: your physical being, your breath, your mind, your intuitive wisdom, and your heart. Use your breath, a bridge between your body and your mind, as a barometer for how you're doing during your pregnancy and labor (just like you do during your yoga practice). If you find yourself holding your breath or losing contact with it altogether, try adding a mantra or a sound to help you follow the inhalations and exhalations up and down your spine. Asking your midwife or partner to breathe with you will also help you stay calmer and more present. Seeing your breath also as the bridge between your heart and your baby will help you remember that the intense sensations you feel during labor are what your baby needs to move out of your womb and into your arms.

Claudia Cummins' Story

Yoga helped me in so many ways during labor and birth. My body was strong, and my understanding of how my body moved—and how it wanted to move—was deep. Many years of cultivating a deeper sense of awareness, as well as a deeper intuitive sense of what felt "right" in my body, my yoga, and my life, helped guide me through the process. I skipped the birthing classes about breathing and positioning the body, figuring my body would know just what to do—and it did. During childbirth, I fell into a very deep chasm and found myself wanting only to listen within. People coaching me from outside, nurses asking me to count breaths, doctors asking me to look in mirrors, and so on felt completely unnecessary and even intrusive. Fortunately, I was surrounded by a team that let me do my own thing. I wouldn't call my experience of childbirth ecstatic, but it was profoundly spiritual—powerful, primal, amazing.

PRANAYAMA

The easiest breathing technique to remember during labor and birthing is called Samavrtti Pranayama (Equal Breathing). Depending on your lung capacity, you simply inhale for 3, 4, or 5 counts and then exhale for the same number of counts. By evening out your breath this way, you can more easily stay in your body and calm your mind at the same time. In the Iyengar tradition, you would do pranayama after asana—that is, after grounding your physical body. Other traditions practice pranayama before a physical practice. Regardless, do them separately; that way you won't be distracted by your body moving around. Pranayama will allow you to dive deeper into your experience and focus on the internal qualities of your body.

STANDING POSES

Standing poses keep your body strong—a strength you'll need during the potentially long hours of labor—and help you to remember to release your pelvis. Do them even when you feel tired, if you can, because they'll show you that you have the stamina and willpower to keep going. Remember, your center of gravity keeps shifting, so do standing poses against the wall or with a chair nearby, just in case. Standing poses can reignite your focus and your confidence and keep your mind engaged—all great tools for preparing for and entering labor and birthing. Some women say that standing poses help them feel the baby more intensely and notice any shifts in his position.

INVERSIONS

Even though the pressure of your baby's head moving into the birth canal might feel only slightly bearable, resist the urge to turn upside down. You want to encourage apana vayu—the downward movement of life force—and not reverse it or slow it down. If you do need a respite, try Adho Mukha Svanasana (Downward-Facing Dog Pose), Uttana Shishosana (Extended Puppy Pose), or even Ardha Adho Mukha Svanasana (Half Downward-Facing Dog Pose) at the wall. Prasarita Padottanasana (Wide-Legged Standing Forward Bend) with your hands on blocks placed fairly far in front of your feet is also a favorite for some women as they approach labor.

SEATED POSES

Practicing poses such as Upavistha Konasana (Wide-Angle Seated Forward Bend), Janu Sisasana (Head-on-Knee Pose), and Baddha Konasana (Bound Angle Pose) with your back against the wall can help you relax and spread your uterine ligaments and pelvic floor muscles, often making labor a little easier.

SQUATS

Either full squats or asymmetrical ones (one knee bent and the other knee down, see pages 163–64) will encourage your pelvic outlet to open and the baby's head to move farther down. Remember, if your baby is not in the right position, you'll want to skip the squats. You don't want these uterine-opening poses to send her farther into your pelvic cavity, where she'll have a much more difficulty maneuvering herself into the right position.

In addition to specific types of poses, returning to the vinyasa concept of arising, abiding, and dissolving may help you ride the waves of intensity and rest in the gaps during your labor. You rise up to meet the sensation (a much gentler term than *contraction*), ride along with it, and then release it, visualizing your baby moving toward the pelvic door. Then you rest in the stillness before another sensation arises.

Yoga always asks us to circle back to our own experience—*What is true for me right now?*—and not allow our minds to get attached to someone else's experience or agenda. Ujjayi Pranayama (Victorious Breathing) can be a gentle way to find some ease within the effort. Research corroborates what we as yoga practitioners already know: smooth, steady breaths that focus on the exhalation can calm the nervous system, produce pain-relieving endorphins, reduce tension in the whole body, and keep our focus internal. The audible vibration in the throat during Ujjayi Pranayama can help keep your attention steady, and by incorporating this breathing into your daily asana practice, you'll have an easier time calling on it during labor. Kundalini yoga master Gurmukh says to put your focus at your third eye (between and slightly above your eyebrows), what she calls the "place of your power."

Birth Wisdom: Coming Back to the Yoga Sutra

How do you know what to do when it comes time to birth your baby? If you've opted for a hospital birth, you may very well have doctors and nurses strongly encouraging medication, and your doula or midwife enthusiastically suggesting alternatives like warm baths, massage, and chanting. Meanwhile, your own mind is questioning your choice to get pregnant in the first place and is convinced that there's no possible way you can endure an hour more of pain. Well before you find yourself in that predicament, spend some time in svadhyaya, communing with the ancient texts (or any writing that helps you feel centered and confident). Make this part of your zwischen, that in-between or "nesting" time most women experience as they move the mind deeper into the body. With so many decisions to make and so much conflicting advice, I found several precepts from the Yoga Sutra quite helpful.

AHIMSA

We all know this cardinal rule of yoga—do no harm. For birthing, this means choosing the kindest, healthiest, and most loving way to give birth, one that supports you and guarantees the safest passage for your baby. We know that events don't always happen the way we envision them, but setting the intention for the most natural birth possible and putting a team together to help that happen may give you peace of mind before labor even starts. You can do this with the understanding that sometimes the least harmful way may end up being a cesarean birth or other forms of medical assistance. It's one thing to be determined to birth your baby naturally but quite another to violate *ahimsa* by being obstinate in the face of medical necessity.

SATYA

This second yama, truthfulness, asks us to be honest with ourselves and with others. Patanjali also says we need to seek inner truth by asking ourselves, *What (not how) am I feeling? What is my experience right now? What am I most afraid of?* If you don't know the answers, you won't know what to ask for, and you'll never know what the real truth was. This also applies to having a baby. Taking time to figure out what lives behind your fears and what you are capable of (on your own and with support) will help you have the most authentic experience, whether you birth at home or in a hospital setting.

ASTEYA

Nonstealing is a funny directive to think about when you're getting ready to give birth. But *asteya* obviously digs deeper than just stealing someone's mat; it reminds you not to let your mind rob you of your focus. Patanjali taught that practicing asteya allows us to live in the present and, most important, to be comfortable with our decisions and the outcomes of those decisions.

One way to practice this principle on your mat is to notice if and when you allow distractions to steal you away from present-moment sensations and even keep you from connecting with your own experience. You might notice what happens on your mat, for instance, when you hold a challenging pose longer than normal. Where does your mind go? Do you stay present to the discomfort, or do you move away from it? This self-awareness is key when you're in labor. Can you keep your focus internal, even when the sensations become almost too intense to bear? Can you reach out for assistance to help you do that? And can you stay true to your own experience, moving and birthing in the best way for you and your baby without being sidelined by other people's expectations?

BRAHMACHARYA

A lot of people interpret this fourth yama as "celibacy or abstinence"— which obviously doesn't pertain to childbirth. Instead, you might look at *brahmacharya* as a way of channeling the passionate energy of making love into birthing your baby. You could also think of it as redirecting your energy back to what is actually happening whenever you get pulled off task.

APARIGRAHA

Traditionally, this ethical precept translates as "nongrasping or nonhoarding," most often showing up as greed or jealousy toward others. In the context of giving birth, *aparigraha* reminds us not to hold on to anything too tightly. For one thing, release those pelvic muscles! But aparigraha also gives you permission to let things unfold, one breath at a time, and to let go of what you think you *should* do so you can focus on what you *can* do. By being more patient, generous, and compassionate with yourself, you may increase the odds of having an experience that leaves you feeling whole and ready to meet and embrace your baby.

CONNECTION AND SUPPORT: YOUR LABOR AND BIRTHING PARTNER SEQUENCES

DE WEST

There will no doubt be times during labor that you'll want to reach out and bring your partner into your experience or ask for help. De West, a pre- and postnatal yoga teacher in Boulder, Colorado, encourages couples to practice these short sequences as often as they like during pregnancy so the poses become second nature to them by the time labor comes along. Partner poses help your partner feel more involved and less anxious and help you both figure out how best to work together while you can still talk and think coherently.

Surya Namaskar (Sun Salutation) Duets

This sequence helps you coordinate your breathing with movements designed to open your hips and lungs. Start with 3 repetitions, moving in unison with your partner. If you're feeling particularly energetic, practice up to 10 of these Surya Namaskars.

Stand in Tadasana (Mountain Pose) with your feet shoulder width apart, facing each other. Bring your hands into prayer position at your heart, and looking directly at each other, inhale deeply. Exhale as you bend down into a partial Malasana (Garland Pose) or squat. Straighten your legs as you inhale, bring your arms up into Urdhva Hastasana (Upward Salute) and look up.

Exhale, extending forward with your arms out to the sides into Ardha Uttanasana (Half Standing Forward Bend); place your hands on blocks to give the baby plenty of room. Bend your knees a little to release your lower back and clasp your hands behind your back. Release the clasp, and inhale as you bring both arms forward toward your partner and hold each other's wrists.

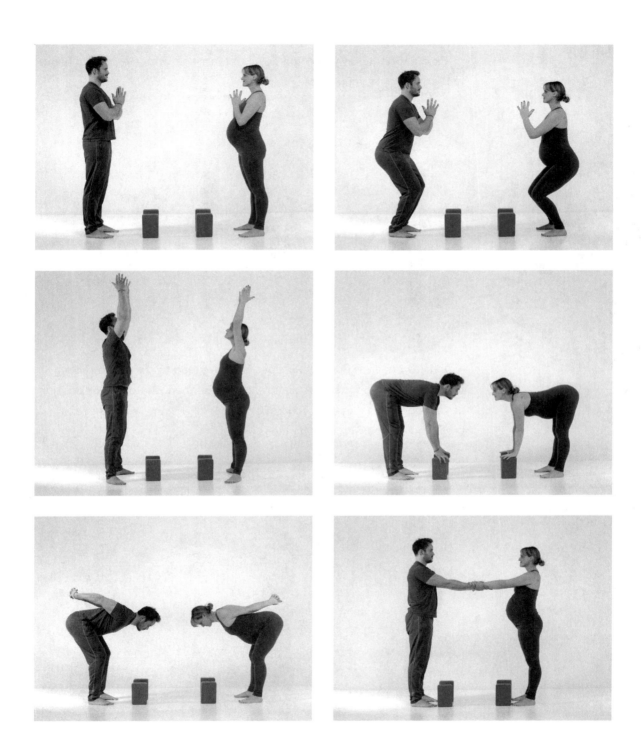

Exhale together as you come down to Malasana, and release your hands to blocks or onto your knees.

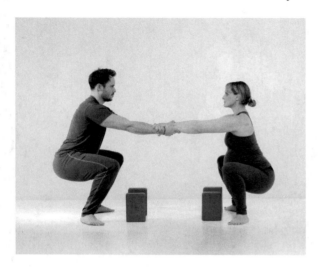
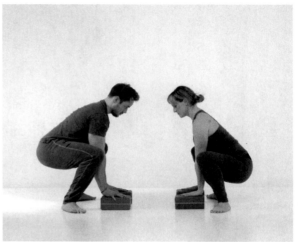

Inhale your arms out to your sides and overhead to come into Urdhva Hastasana. On your next exhalation, bring your hands into prayer position at your heart and remain in Tadasana for several breaths, matching your breathing rhythm with your partner's.

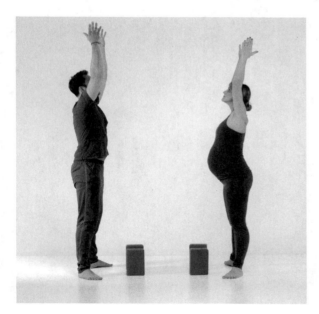
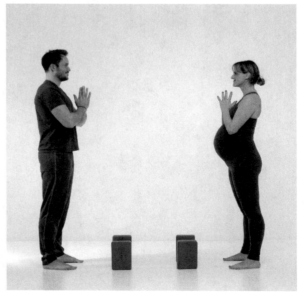

Partner Squatting Vinyasa

Practicing this sequence before you go into active labor will help your partner know what type of touch and pressure you like and need (which, of course, may change once labor starts).

Position a chair on a sticky mat, cover the hard edge of the seat with a blanket, and ask your partner to sit down. Come into Malasana (Garland Pose) or full squat facing away from the chair, using any props you need (a block or bolster to sit on, for example), and lean into your partner for support. Your partner's forearms should be under your armpits to lift you slightly, creating space in your side waist, lungs, and diaphragm and also creating more space for your baby. This squatting position will be home base for this sequence. Breathe here for 5 to 8 long, smooth Ujjayi breaths.

When you're ready to move, ask your partner to assist you with a gentle push away from the chair and onto your hands and knees. From all fours, place your left foot on the ground to your left, across from your right knee, and come into an asymmetrical squat with your hands still on the floor.

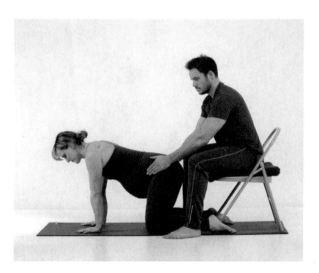

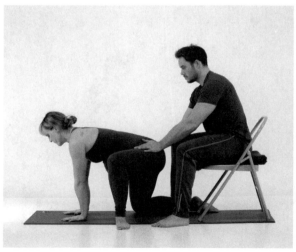

Now begin to move your pelvis in whatever way feels good—rocking from side to side, moving in circles, tilting and tucking—while your partner gently performs the "double hip squeeze," pressing your hips toward the midline to release and support your pelvis. Move for several breaths or as long as it feels good.

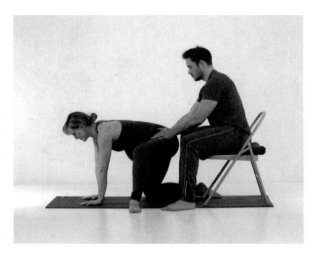 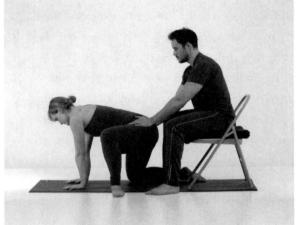

Come back to your hands and knees, with your knees positioned slightly wider than hip-width apart. Continue to do pelvic movements and rocking. Your partner's loving hands can support your pelvis in rhythm with your movements.

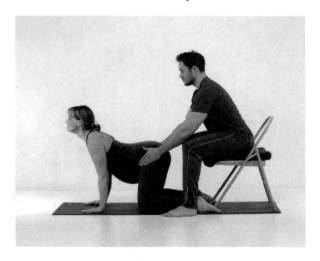 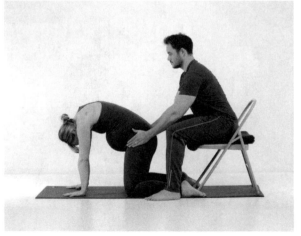

Whenever you're ready, push back into Balasana (Child's Pose) with the support of your partner, and breathe deeply. Your partner can rub your back or press downward from the top of your buttocks toward your heels, whichever works for you. When you're ready, return to all fours and repeat the sequence on the other side.

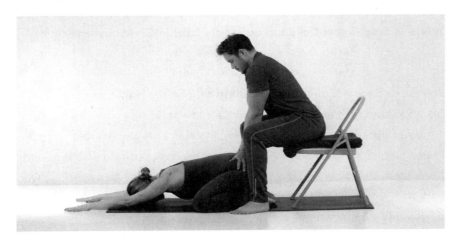

When you come out of Balasana, move back into Malasana with your partner in the chair for support. This time your partner can gently massage your jaw, release any tension in your shoulders, and encourage you to lean back while relaxing and reminding you what a beautiful and amazing woman you are.

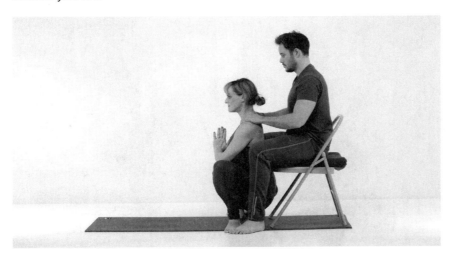

FLOWING WITH THE BREATH: SOUND AND MOVEMENT FOR LABOR AND BIRTH

DE WEST

Doing asana in concert with deep, guttural sounds can help you focus your attention deep in your belly and assist your baby in a safe outward journey.

Vajrasana Surya Namaskar (Kneeling Sun Salutation)

From Vajrasana (Thunderbolt Pose), inhale as you bring your arms out to the sides and overhead, lifting your hips to stand on your knees.

With a humming exhalation, release your arms back down to your hips and lower your sitting bones back onto your heels. Continue this mini vinyasa for 8 to 12 repetitions, feeling the vibrations of the audible exhalation deep in your belly.

BENEFITS: These movements strengthen your legs and spine, release your shoulders, and open your chest.

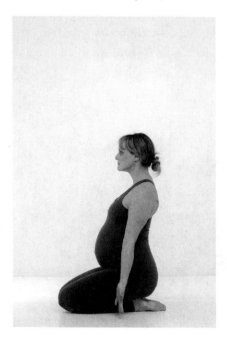 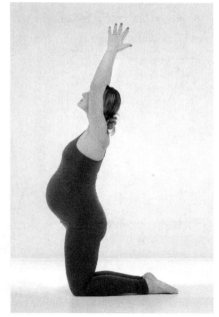

Humming Dolphin

Come onto your hands and knees with your shoulders over your wrists and your knees slightly wider than hip-width apart. Draw your belly in ever so slightly to protect your lower back. As you inhale, arch your back, lift your face, and imagine you're a dolphin lifting your tail to the sky. Exhale as you lower your imaginary dolphin tail into the water, rounding your spine.

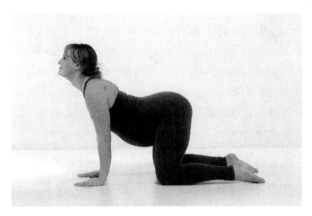 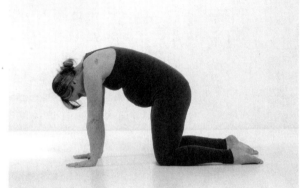

Make a low, soft humming sound during the exhalation. Continue this pattern for 8 to 10 repetitions, blending one movement and breath into the next.

NOTE: The dolphin imagery may help you find the fluid movement and rhythm of being in water. Imagine your baby riding her own waves.

BENEFITS: During the early stages of labor, this mini vinyasa may help move the baby away from your back and relieve pressure on your bladder.

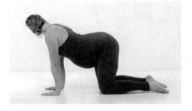

Hissing Fish

Staying on your hands and knees, move your imaginary fish tail to the right as you inhale and look over your right shoulder. Part your lips and exhale back to center, making a hissing sound—as if you were going to say, "Sit." Inhale your tail to the left while you look left. Exhale as you hiss and move back to center. Repeat this movement pattern 8 to 10 times.

BENEFITS: Moving your pelvis through a variety of positions can free up any tension or holding. Hissing is a great way to relax your mouth, the back of your throat, your pelvic floor, and your whole nervous system.

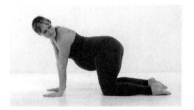

Mama Salutes with Sound

This gentle vinyasa may feel grounding and energizing during the very early stages of labor, when you can still move around relatively easily. With every exhalation, open your mouth, keep your face relaxed, and let out an easy "aah" sound. The more you can soften your throat, eyes, and face, the easier it will be to soften and release your pelvic muscles.

Stand in Tadasana (Mountain Pose) with your feet parallel and mat-width apart and your hands in prayer at your heart. Inhale as you raise your arms out to the sides and over your head into Urdhva Hastasana (Upward Salute). Exhale an "aah" as you extend forward, chest lifted, into Uttanasana (Standing Forward Bend), placing your hands on the blocks in front of you. Release your head and neck. As you inhale, bring your chest forward and lift your chin a bit into Ardha Uttanasana. On an exhalation,

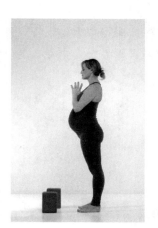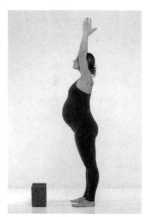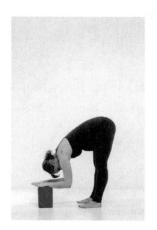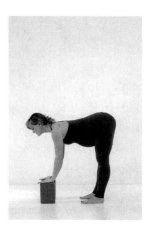

move your blocks back between your feet and step your right leg back into High Lunge, keeping your left knee over your ankle. Draw your hips in toward one another so you don't overstretch, but you should still feel that you're releasing your inner thigh and groin muscles.

Drop your right knee to the floor, and move your left knee back so you are on all fours with your hips slightly wider than your knees. Keep your blocks nearby. Inhale as you bring your chest forward and your tailbone up toward the ceiling in Cat/Cow Pose. Exhale an "aah," round your spine, and drop your tailbone toward the floor.

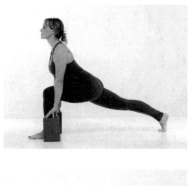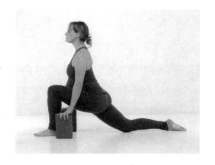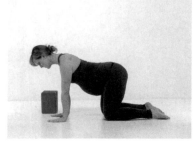

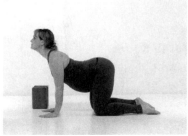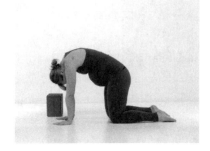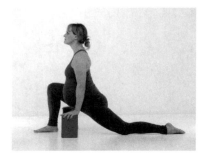

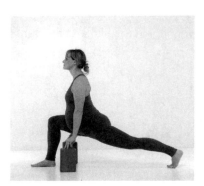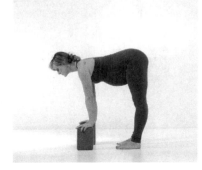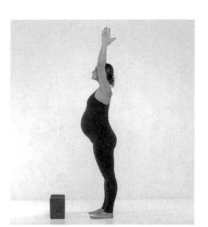

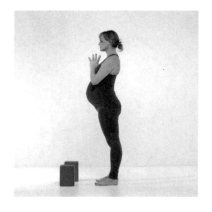

Inhale your right foot forward into Anjaneyasana (Low Lunge), placing your hands on your blocks. Make sure your right foot is all the way over toward the outside edge of your mat to create more space for your belly. Then lift your left leg behind you into High Lunge. When you're ready, exhale your left foot forward, then inhale as you come up into Ardha Uttanasana (Half Standing Forward Bend). Exhale and drop your head without collapsing your chest. Bending your knees a little, inhale and reach your arms out to the sides and overhead as you come to standing. Exhale your hands to prayer position at your heart and rest in Tadasana. Repeat the sequence on the opposite side.

NOTE: Make the sounds low and guttural to bring the vibration down into your belly and encourage apana vayu.

BENEFITS: These salutes help move energy downward, especially during the "aah" of each exhalation, and encourage your baby to move deeper into position.

CAUTION: Don't practice Mama Salutes if you feel tired or you have progressed to active labor.

Virabhadrasana I (Warrior I Pose) Flow with Sound

If Mama Salutes are too energetic, you may prefer this sequence, which calls on the strength of your legs and the muscles between your shoulder blades.

Begin in Tadasana (Mountain Pose) and step your left foot behind you to prepare for Virabhadrasana I. Keep both legs straight. If you feel unstable, either shorten your stance or move your right foot a little to the right.

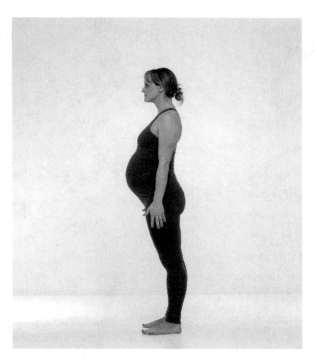
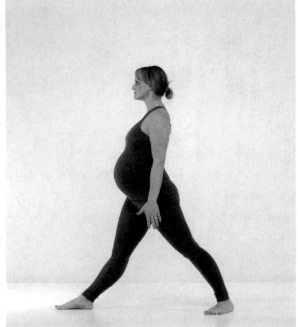

Inhale as you bring your arms overhead into Urdhva Hastasana (Upward Salute). As you exhale, bend your right knee and pull your elbows down until your upper arms are parallel to the ground, forming cactus arms; stick out your tongue and push the exhalation out, making a louder "aah" sound. Inhale again, straighten your right knee, and lift your arms back overhead. Exhale and, keeping your legs straight, bring your arms down by your sides. Do this sequence 4 to 6 times, then reverse legs and repeat.

BENEFITS: Your chest will feel open, and the upward movement of your arms will bring more space into the sides of your waist, making it easier for you to breathe.

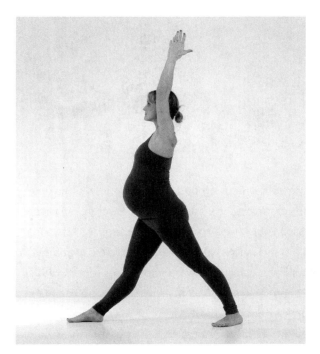 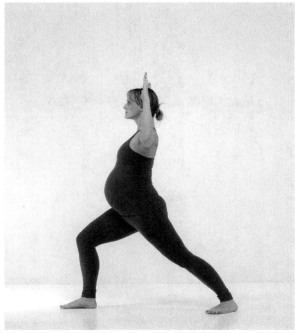

Seated Flow—Moaning

Sit on a folded blanket with your back against a wall and your legs stretched out in front of you in a gentle Upavistha Konasana (Wide-Angle Seated Pose). Your feet should be a comfortable distance apart, but not wide enough to feel any pressure on your pubic bone. Inhale and point your toes; exhale and draw your toes back. Make a moaning sound with each exhalation. It can be loud or soft, but let the sound come from deep in your pelvis.

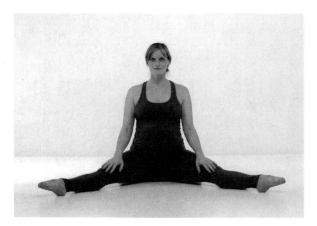

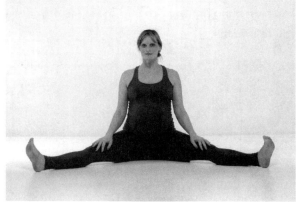

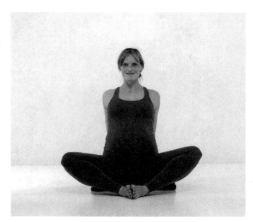

Continue your breathing pattern and circle your ankles (a few times clockwise, then a few times counterclockwise). Reach behind your knees and guide your legs into Baddha Konasana (Bound Angle Pose). Press your heels together and let your thighs stretch toward your knees, opening your pelvis and inner thighs. Place your hands behind you and press them into the floor to lift your ribs off your pelvis, creating a little more space. Let your breath be soft, focusing on the space right below your breastbone where your rib cage starts to open. Hold here for 4 to 6 breaths.

De's Story

At thirty-six weeks, my water broke. No contractions or other signs of labor were present, so I decided to drive home and check in with my support team. By the time I got home, I was leaking amniotic fluid all over. I called my doula, who suggested I check in with my doctor; my doctor suggested I check into the hospital. I laughed. "No, I need to eat, pack, connect with my husband, and write my birth plan!"

My husband and I headed to my acupuncturist, David, who put me in a dark, quiet room. With needles in my back and electric stimulation on the needles, David fed me herbs by the dropperful as I started to go inward. I focused on relaxing, feeling my breath and connecting with my baby.

I visualized my cervix opening to a ten-centimeter circle mandala. I visualized a pillar of light from my head to my pelvic floor, and I calmed my fear of the unknown. I mentally focused my attention inward to what I wanted to happen next. I imagined letting go of the list of things I was still holding on to: the yoga class I was supposed to be teaching, the baby's room that wasn't done, the work I would have to miss, the unfinished birth plan, and the baby shower that was scheduled in two days. Soon after my letting-go meditation, I started having contractions and headed home to labor.

During my seven-hour labor, I made a lot of noise. I moaned softly and loudly; I chanted OM and yelled, "ah," and my support team sounded with me, which was a powerful choir. Sounding helped me manage my pain, connect with the contractions, and ride the waves of my labor. An hour after we got to the hospital I was fully dilated, and after two hours of pushing, my daughter Anahata was born. I believe the messages we send ourselves do matter. I believe our breath is a powerful carrier of those messages. I also believe making sound can release energy and send messages through the vibration of our being.

Use your hands again to move your legs back into Upavistha Konasana. Be careful not to overstretch. Sit up tall, lifting your spine. Hold here for 4 to 6 breaths. Come into Sukhasana (Easy Seated Pose) as you draw your attention inward and focus on keeping your breath steady. Visualize the exhalation moving down into your pelvic area and farther to your pelvic floor. Hold here for 6 to 8 breaths.

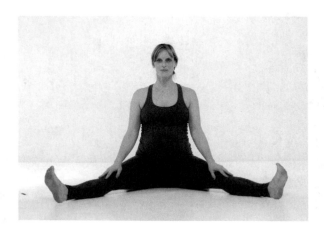 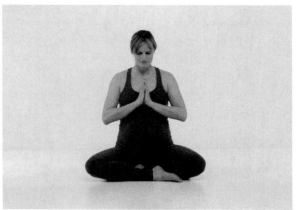

CAUTION: Avoid folding forward in this position. A forward bending movement with your legs stretched wide can destabilize your pelvis and misalign your pubis.

BENEFITS: Baddha Konasana and Upavistha Konasana are especially beneficial because they help broaden your pelvic area and dilate your cervix.

How to Breathe
When Labor Becomes Intense

• Be gentle with your breathing. Don't force the inhalation or press down on the exhalation. Allow the rhythm of your breath to flow as freely as you can.

• When you have trouble finding your rhythm, try counting the duration of the inhalation and exhalation (either keeping them equal—4 counts in, 4 counts out—or drawing out the exhalation a little longer than the inhalation).

• Ask your midwife or partner to do conscious breathing so you can follow along. Taking time before labor to practice together will help your support person know what breathing techniques work best for you.

• If you need to recommit to your breathing, Viloma Pranayama I (Interval Breathing I) without retention can help. The focus of this three-part breath should be on the inhalation. Inhale to your navel and pause; take the inhalation up to your rib cage and pause; then continue the inhalation all the way to your collarbones. Pause and let the air all the way out in one smooth exhalation. Repeat this pranayama 5 to 7 times before returning to your normal breathing pattern.

• Adding sound to your breathing, especially the exhalation, also helps you find your breath again. Niika Quistgard's toning advice on pages 146–47 is great; De West's Flowing with the Breath sequence (page 166) also works well.

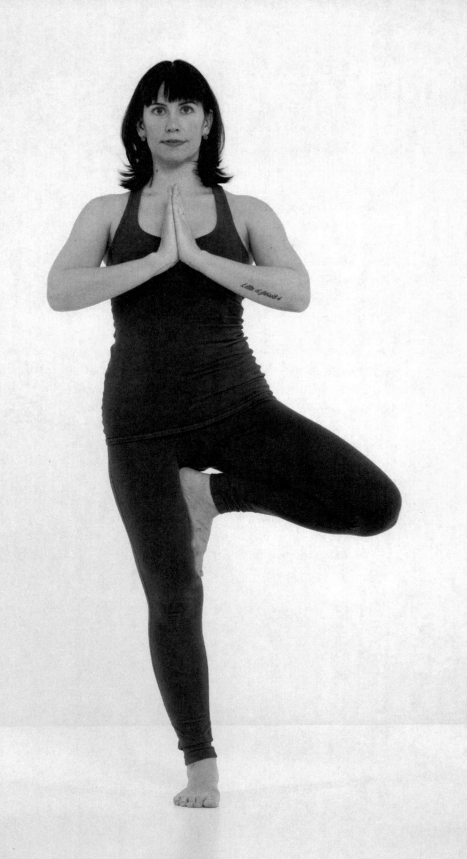

6.

FOURTH TRIMESTER

Welcoming Baby Home
From Birth to Twelve Weeks

Sequences by Dustienne Miller
and Kate Hanley

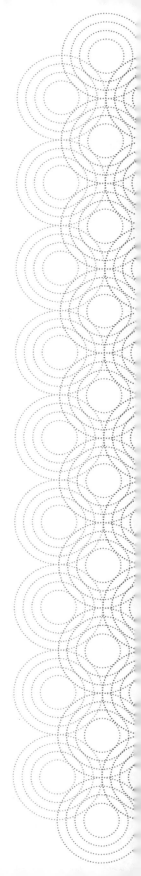

No one needs to tell you that giving birth requires tremendous physical and emotional strength—some even say it's more difficult than running a marathon, and for most women it certainly takes longer. Regardless of whether your experience went according to your birth plan, you did it. You gave birth to your baby—what could be more awesome than that? How you choose to spend these next few months will influence your physical and mental well-being for years to come, which will in turn fortify you with the strength and patience you need to care for yourself and your child.

Most yoga mamas want to know how quickly they can resume their yoga practice. Often the hidden concern behind that question is "how quickly will I get my body back?" In fact, I would like to suggest that the question become "How can I rebuild my yoga practice in a way that creates a healthy postnatal body and a peaceful mind?" and that the correct answer be "from the ground up, mindfully and patiently." Because so much happens in this "fourth trimester," I think it'll help to break things down in stages. Let's start by exploring what's happening in your body now that you've given birth. Then we can examine some of the challenges you may be facing and how yoga can hopefully mitigate them. We'll devote a large part of this chapter on how to get both your practice and your body back safely. Of course, just when you're ready to hit the mat in full-on "I'm back" mode, you'll find you have no time of your own. So, in an effort not to leave you stranded, we'll wrap up with some good ways of sneaking in a daily practice.

Establishing the Love Connection

Both Western and ayurvedic doctors agree that baby should stay as close to his mama as possible during the first three months of life. In this "fourth trimester" you and your baby are still inexorably linked—in fact, many midwives actually use the term *motherbaby* to describe this interconnected state—and are trying to find your way in the world. It's good to remember that your little one has just emerged from a dark, warm, safe place into a brighter, louder, colder environment—especially if you've given birth in a hospital setting. Immediately putting him on your bare chest (without cleaning him up or swaddling him) in a warm, dimly lit room, with a light blanket over the two of you will help that transition and keep the hormones of attachment strong.

Continue skin-to-skin contact as long as possible and whenever you can; your partner can do that too, creating a wonderful opportunity for the two of them to bond while you take a little time for yourself. To comfort your baby, play the same soft music he enjoyed in utero; swaddle him; and sing, chant, sway, and rock.

As my grandmother always said, you can't spoil a baby with too much love. Your job right now is to help your baby transition from womb to room as gently and lovingly as you can. For many families, that means co-sleeping, nursing on demand, and swaddling or carrying the baby in a sling or front pack. Studies now show that your hugs, cuddles, kisses, coos, and massages have immediate and long-lasting benefits for your baby—and for you—and will help him be better able to handle all the new world stressors coming his way. Try not to rush this time of connection. Staying with whatever is happening as it happens will help you slowly transition into the rest of your life, whatever that might mean for you, and will soften any feelings of fear, resentment, or impatience that may surface.

Whenever you feel rushed, stressed, or overwhelmed, especially during these first few months, return to your breathing practices. Belly Breathing, Nadi Shodhana (Alternate Nostril Breathing), and Ujjayi Pranayama (Victorious Breath) will help you slow down and stay in the moment. In fact, you can begin gentle pranayama practices as soon after giving birth as you'd like. As we'll discuss later in this chapter, pranayama is a gentle yet powerful way to begin to knit things back together.

The Inside Scoop

You may be basking in post-birth bliss now, which is driven by hormones like everything else that's happened to you over the last nine months. Physiologically, that "ecstatic cocktail" of hormones that allowed you to birth your baby (oxytocin, beta-endorphins, and prolactin) is still in abundance, especially if you had a natural childbirth experience, ensuring that your transition into motherhood is as stress-free and loving as possible. According to Sarah Buckley, MD, those extra-high levels of hormones play a role in encouraging us to be "hopelessly devoted" to our babies and have plenty of energy and a singular focus despite our lack of sleep. Although there's no medical evidence that the hormones remain in that intensified state longer than a few hours, some women and their partners experience a rush of energy and a sense of euphoria that lasts much longer than logic would dictate—even a couple of weeks. According to Dr. Buckley, there appears to be a reorganization of the brain in these hormonal areas that throws the switch on instinctive mothering. She says that women who have given birth more than once have more oxytocin in their system, which often makes subsequent births easier and switches the mothering instinct on faster.

The increase of these hormones doesn't happen if you've had synthetic oxytocin to jump-start labor, an epidural for pain, or a cesarean birth, which may make the first couple of postpartum weeks more difficult than you expected. That's because cesarean births and other medical procedures often bring pretty intense post-birthing pains and require a longer recovery time. And, let's get real: it's hard to give anyone, including your baby, your undivided, loving attention when your whole body hurts or you're on pain medication. But that doesn't mean your mother-baby bonding can't be strong and meaningful. Nature provides other opportunities to keep those bonding hormones pumping and the mother-baby connection strong: breastfeeding, which Dr. Buckley calls Nature's back-up plan; and skin-to-skin contact, which a 2012 study from St. Francis Xavier University found helps reduce postpartum depression and physiological stress. Another study published in 2013 in *International Breastfeed Journal* also noted that skin-to-skin contact—holding your naked baby against your naked chest—while breastfeeding has a calming effect on babies who have difficulty latching on to their mothers' nipples and helps them nurse more effectively.

Reaching out to friends and family provides yet another way to increase oxytocin and help you transition into motherhood. In a June, 2013 TED talk in Edinburgh, Kelly McGonigal, PhD, a health psychologist and lecturer at Stanford University, said that when oxytocin is released it "motivates you to seek support, nudging you to tell someone how you feel," instead of internalizing everything. According to McGonigal, the more you reach out, the more oxytocin is released, which helps you trust your ability to handle life's challenges "knowing you don't have to face them alone." Allowing friends and family to cook meals, tidy up, do laundry, walk your baby while you sleep, take your other children on an outing, give you a soothing massage—whatever *you* need—will help you recover faster and will also give you uninterrupted quiet time with your baby so you won't feel torn between bonding with her and getting things done. The less stressed you are, the easier the transition will be for both of you.

The ayurvedic name for this hormonal-rich state of altered awareness is *sutaka*. Sutaka, which means "charioteer or one who transports precious cargo" begins during labor and birth and refers to that altered state when a woman puts her logical, neocortex brain on hold and allows the primordial mammalian brain to take over and shepherd her baby into the world. Ayurvedic specialist Claudia Welch, PhD, says during postpartum sutaka, a mother may experience a strong feeling of connection with and acceptance of her own needs and those of her baby, less anxiety over little things, deep relaxation and a feeling that "all's right with the world." Even lovelier, she says, sutaka also touches those present at the birth of your child—your partner, midwife, or any family members—even without the benefit of birthing hormones.

Fourth Trimester Challenges

For at least the first couple of weeks after you've given birth, yoga's "listen to your body" imperative will take on a heightened sense of urgency. In fact, your body with its inflamed tissues, enormous breasts, and sore muscles is positively yelling at you. You're probably exhausted (especially if this pregnancy was your first) and quite possibly overwhelmed and overloaded. On top of all that, you may be trying to figure out how to nurse, when to sleep, what to eat, and why you alternately can't stop crying and smiling uncontrollably. Even if none of this is your experience and you feel fabulous, your body needs time to readjust and recover. The practices and rituals you create now should support your body's healing journey and help you sort through and honor your physical limitations and your emotions as they present themselves. And, for heaven's sake, don't be shy. Speak up and ask for what you need—whether it's emotional, physical, practical, or all of the above.

UTERINE CONTRACTIONS

Just when you thought your contractions were over, they're back—at least for another couple weeks, particularly when you nurse. Luckily they won't be nearly as intense as during labor. Welcome them. They exist, courtesy of the ever-present hormone oxytocin, to shrink your uterus back to its normal size and shape. The more you nurse, the faster your uterus will contract. Massaging your uterus will lessen the intensity of these pains and so will relaxing into any restorative yoga poses that give your uterus a bit of a lift and help stop your postpartum bleeding a little sooner, like Supta Virasana (Reclining Hero Pose) fully supported with bolsters and blankets. You may prefer pressure against your abdomen instead and enjoy gently pressing a bolster or pillow against your belly in Balasana (Child's Pose) or Paschimottanasana (Seated Forward Bend).

TEARS OR STITCHES

If you tore giving birth and needed stitches, or if you had an episiotomy, you may not want to do much that stretches or pulls. My daughter Megan, who had a relatively quick natural childbirth, said the most painful part of the whole experience was mending from the tear she experienced while pushing—it stung like crazy and then itched impossibly. She didn't feel like doing any physical asanas until all that was over. If you've had a cesarean birth, you'll want to wait until the wound has healed, usually about six to eight weeks.

THE BABY BLUES: A REAL PERSPECTIVE ON POSTPARTUM DEPRESSION

If I'm supposed to be so in love with my baby, why am I crying all the time? It's only been four days . . . but it feels like forever. Have I failed as a mother? At some point in their postnatal journey, most women ask such questions, so if these could be your anguished queries, please know that you haven't failed and you are certainly not alone. Just as postnatal bliss can raise you up into a crazy, euphoric state, the baby blues can cause everything to come crashing back down. Higher than imaginable one moment, lower than low the next—both feelings are a bit disconcerting and utterly normal. The baby blues, which some experts say at least 80 percent of women experience (even midwives, doulas, and yoga teachers!), can come on a few days after giving birth and last a couple weeks, causing you to feel alternately anxious and depressed.

Postpartum depression (PPD), on the other hand, is a bit more severe. It affects anywhere from 5 to 20 percent of new mothers and can show up anytime after you've given birth—but usually within the first year—and be hard to shake. Some PPD symptoms include loss of appetite and difficulty bonding with your baby, trouble sleeping, nightmares, bizarre thoughts, withdrawal from your friends and family, and feelings of shame and inadequacy.

Several factors conspire to bring you down, foremost among them being hormones. Shortly after giving birth your estrogen and progesterone plummet and your thyroid hormones take a tumble as well, all of which can leave you feeling sluggish and blue. According to Mayo Clinic, changes in your blood pressure, immune system function, and metabolism can also contribute to depression. Not getting enough sleep or enough emotional support makes even the simplest things seem insurmountable. Your breasts hurt and leak; you feel dumpy; all your baby seems to do is cry and want to nurse; you're exhausted; and your whole support team has gone back to normal life. And, on top of everything else, you may feel like you've lost your identity and given up any sense of independence.

If your postpartum depression doesn't improve after three weeks, you can't seem to find a way out of it, or (more important) you're afraid you'll hurt your baby or yourself, please seek help from a qualified therapist right away.

Conscious lifestyle changes, plus yoga and pranayama can often make you feel better faster. First of all, be gentle with yourself. Just because you are suffering does not mean you are a bad mother, nor does it mean that you don't love your baby or that you'll always feel like this. A bout of the baby blues or postpartum depression is a great time to remember two important teachings of yoga practice: self-reflection without judgment and all things arise, abide, and (fortunately) dissolve. In the meantime, there are a few practical things you can do that may lift you up and out of the blues.

- Focus on anything that will make you feel better, such as sleep and food. It's hard to heal when you can't sleep and neglect your own basic needs. And we know that lack of sleep makes everything appear much worse.
- Do yoga. Whether or not you've healed enough to resume your pre-pregnancy routine, practicing restorative poses and pranayama may help center you and get you back into your body. It may also help you understand that you are not your depression and that this, too, shall pass.
- Reach out for help. No one ever said having a new baby would be easy, nor were you meant to do this all by yourself. So, don't

be afraid or ashamed to ask for what you need; it really does take a village! When my friend Lesli had twins and was completely overwhelmed, a bunch of us organized a meal team (each taking on one day's worth of meals that also yielded leftovers). A massage therapist friend gave the new mama a weekly treatment at home and her sister made it a point to take the twins on daily walks so Lesli could eat a meal in silence, take an uninterrupted shower, put on real clothes, and even blow-dry her hair. Not only can connecting with supportive, loving friends and family members make you feel better, it actually has a positive neurological effect on your body by raising levels of oxytocin (the feel-good hormone) and making you feel stronger and more capable. In fact, as Kelly McGonigal says, the more you reach out the more apt you are to trust your own abilities.

◆ Breastfeed. For many women, nursing gives them a loving connection with their baby that produces a sense of calm for both. Also, breastfeeding increases oxytocin and can make you feel better. If you and your baby are having trouble getting the feeding rhythm down, you might want to contact a lactation consultant or open up to a friend who's more experienced. Of course, if your baby is nursing every two hours, even at night, you may not feel all that loving toward her. Consider pumping and ask your partner to take over a few night feedings so you can get the sleep you need.

◆ Get out of the house. Going outside—even if you just walk around the block—helps. Give yourself a change of scenery, feel the sun (or even rain or snow!) on your skin, and breathe it all in. Another friend told me she made a point every day, no matter how low she felt, to shower, get dressed, and go somewhere.

◆ Take one step, no matter how small. Several years ago, an executive vice president at Google told me that he commits to two minutes of meditation or yoga every day. Sometimes those two minutes turn into 15 or 20; sometimes he manages to meditate *and* do yoga. But the duration or amount doesn't matter. What does matter, he says, is that he knows he always has time to do something for two minutes. What can you do for two or maybe five minutes each day that will make you feel better?

• Count your blessings. A simple practice of writing down—or mentally saying—what you're grateful for can sometimes shift your mood.

• Be with other moms. As soon as you feel up to going out, join a moms' group or reconnect with your friends who have babies or little kids. Being with others who've had similar experiences will help you realize you're not crazy or as isolated as you sometimes feel, and other women may be able to share what has worked for them.

Sometimes PPD can be the result of feeling guilty, sad, disappointed, or angry that your birthing experience did not go according to plan. Ginny Hendricksen, a ballet dancer with Ballet Flanders in Belgium, said her depression came from feeling she had missed out on the natural childbirth experience she had so looked forward to. "I practiced hypno-birthing meditation right up to the day I went into labor, and I had a birth plan that didn't include any medication," she says. What she got was the exact opposite—an emergency cesarean birth three weeks early without the support of her husband, who was out of town. Ginny said it helped her heal to focus on "the miracle of having a small human who needed me and being thankful for modern medicine that ending up keeping us both alive." Some women find release and relief from being able to talk about their disappointment or feelings of failure. Many midwives and doulas are trained in what they call birth-reclaiming practices.

How Yoga Can Help

While the gentle sequences that Dustienne provides in this chapter—with their focus on Belly Breathing—will help you get back into your body in a way that can soothe and support you, the addition of pranayama, asana, and mantra meditation may alleviate mild postpartum depression.

EMPHASIZE THE INHALATION

Pranayama techniques that focus on the inhalation and expansion of your ribcage and chest can increase your energy and wake up your nervous system. Practice Viloma Pranayama I (Interval Breathing I)—with an emphasis on the inhalation—either sitting with your eyes closed or lying in a restorative pose like Viparita Karani (Legs up the Wall pose): Inhale to your navel and pause; take the inhalation up to your ribcage and pause; and then continue the inhalation all the way to your collarbones. Pause and let the air all the way out in one smooth exhalation.

MOVE INTO YOUR BODY

If you've stopped bleeding (or your cesarean incisions have healed), and your body feels up to it, you can start exploring some gentle posture- and mood-improving poses. Tadasana (Mountain Pose), Vrksasana (Tree Pose), and Urdhva Hastasana (Upward Salute) from Dustienne's Standing Sequence will get your blood flowing and your energy rising. Do these poses at the wall if you don't feel strong enough to stand on your own two feet quite yet, or enlist the help of a partner.

CHANT YOUR FAVORITE MANTRA

Sometimes it's hard to access the breath or practice asana when your heart's not in it. When that happens, try adding sound to your experience to keep you focused. Ujjayi Pranayama (Victorious Breath), with its soft ocean sound, is a lovely way to move the inhalation up into spaces it may be reluctant to inhabit and to usher the exhalation out of your body completely. Chanting OM or a simple mantra such as SO-HUM also encourages the breath to expand your ribcage and chest wall and then to fully release everything. I find this practice quite energizing and effective, especially when I add an emotional element to it. I inhale a joyful memory and exhale the doldrums out of my body, which makes me feel better.

SIGN UP FOR A POSTNATAL YOGA CLASS

Joining a moms-and-babies yoga class is a great way to get out of the house and do something fun and energizing with your little one.

Postnatal yoga classes give yoga mamas an opportunity to share stories and advice, which can put many things into perspective. They offer a healing experience for your body and your emotions and give you a chance to spend time with your baby in the company of others. Many postnatal yoga teachers are also doulas or midwives, so they can be excellent resources for after-birth advice.

Your Yoga Practice: The Fourth Trimester

How should you approach your practice after birthing your baby? When can you get back to your mat in earnest? There's no iron-clad rule about what to do when—after you've stopped bleeding, of course, and have begun to feel more like yourself. Every woman has a different experience. Every pregnancy and every postpartum adventure is unique. Some women are ready three weeks after giving birth; others take their time and may not want to resume the pre-baby routine for several months (if ever). Most ayurvedic physicians caution not to do much except restorative poses, visualizations, and gentle pranayama for at least three months; some teachers even say you shouldn't engage in a more vigorous practice until you stop nursing. I say check in with your body and ask the questions *how are you doing?* and *what do you need?* before deciding your course of action. You've just spent the last nine months (and probably years before that) connecting pretty deeply with your body, your breath, and your mind. You probably learned to ascertain what feels good and what doesn't, what you need and what doesn't really work for you (and now your baby). Approach your postpartum decisions the same way. Although my usual "it depends" answer still stands, please don't rush.

For the first two to three weeks or so, have your practice be anything that allows you to rest, rebalance, replenish, and reconnect with your baby, your own body, and your partner. You can certainly do simple pranayamas and Savasana as soon as you want. As you get a little more energy, some gentle yoga that focuses on your pelvic floor, as well as additional pranayama techniques, should feel soothing and healing. The bottom line: be patient. Doing yoga that supports and heals your tissues, rebalances your prana (life force), and moves you gently back into stasis—as opposed to jumping right into your pre-pregnancy routine—will let you get the most benefit from your practice and emerge physically stronger, mentally clearer, and emotionally more present.

When my second child was born, I committed to giving myself six weeks with no agenda, no timetable, and no goals, which helped me immensely. My practice was simply to feed, love, and care for my daughter and to take the time to discover what it meant to be her mother. I wanted to learn how to give my baby and my older daughter what they needed and to honor and support myself sufficiently so that their needs didn't overwhelm mine. Gentle pranayama, Savasana, sleep, restorative poses, and the famous Ram Dass mantra BE HERE NOW sustained me, especially for the first two or three weeks. I found this yogic prescription to be invaluable as I attempted to rebalance my body's "systems"—my digestive, endocrine, and nervous systems, in particular—and prepared to knit things back together.

Once you feel ready, whether four weeks or six months have passed, you can begin to shift your practice to create a foundation of connection and stability. All through your pregnancy, you focused on poses that created space for your baby, broadened your hips, and moved the energy downward. Now, you'll want to concentrate on knitting everything back together, encouraging your uterus to move back into place and realigning your posture. Keep in mind that your joints are probably still somewhat hypermobile (the hormone relaxin stays relatively high for several months after you give birth), so be extra careful not to overstretch. In order for your practice to serve your body, and not harm it unwittingly, you'll need to keep a few important rules in mind.

- Don't try to go beyond what feels comfortable. This is no time to "get better at" or go deeper into poses.
- Don't hold on too tightly to one way of doing things. Be flexible enough to modify poses according to your energy level, the way your body feels, the amount of sleep you've gotten, your mood, and what kind of time you can carve out for yourself.

- Avoid energizing breathing practices like Kapalabhati Pranayama (Breath of Fire), which sometimes causes your pelvic floor and your oblique abdominals to contract, potentially increasing prolapse problems.
- Avoid any poses that engage your superficial abdominal muscles (the six-pack abs)—at least for the first two or three months. That means no crunches, no Pilates-style sit-ups, and no moves that push against the abdominal wall.
- Avoid poses that encourage asymmetrical movement until your pelvic floor is stronger, including lunges, Utthita Trikonasana (Extended Triangle Pose), Utthita Parsvakonasana (Extended Side-Angle Pose), and Janu Sirsasana (Head-to-Knee Pose).
- Focus on poses that gently draw energy (and your muscles) in and up. (See Dustienne's Gravity-Eliminating Flow Practice on page 193).
- Avoid unsupported poses that put too much pressure on your groin for the first two months. These include Supta Baddha Konasana (Reclining Bound Angle Pose), Baddha Konasana (Bound Angle Pose), and Upavistha Konasana (Wide-Angle Seated Pose).

Getting Your Body Back

Most women are eager to shed their post-birth excess and start wearing their old clothes again. You may feel that way, too. I certainly did. For some reason, when I gave birth to my older daughter, I packed my skinny jeans and a little T-shirt because I thought I could wear my regular clothes home from the birthing center. My mother told me she actually did. Of course, she neglected to add that she had spent two weeks in the hospital and favored relatively baggy clothes back then. I was horrified to discover that I still looked pregnant and that I could lift up my belly and let it flop against my body. Needless to say, I shelved my skinny jeans for a few more months. To comfort myself, I decided that I would "loan" my body to my baby girl, focusing on and celebrating its ability to feed and comfort her and giving it the time and nonjudgmental attention it needed to do that.

What does it mean to "get your body back"? Do you hope you'll look the same as you did ten, eleven, or twelve months ago? That may happen a few months (or a year) down the road, but what if it doesn't? Can you be okay with that? I think it does help to remind yourself that the body you have right now is serving you and your baby just fine. It's exactly what, where, and how it needs to be. It also helps to remember that your body has a lot to figure out right now. Early on in this fourth trimester, your breasts are working on regulating the flow of milk so your baby gets the right amount for her to grow, your tissues are healing, and your uterus is shrinking back to its pre-pregnancy size. Treat your body with the generosity and patience it deserves, and tailor your activities (including yoga and meditation) to focus on resting, nourishing, and healing as well as building strength and finding balance.

Both ayurvedic physicians and Western physical therapists agree that the body has the best chance at returning to its pre-birth shape and strength if you take things slowly. There'll be plenty of time to reinvigorate your six-pack abs and pour yourself into those skinny jeans. But in order to ensure that your body is fit and healthy for the long haul, experts recommend that you heal the tissues first and then start from the bottom (the pelvic floor) up to connect and strengthen.

HEALING THE TISSUES

Pregnancy, labor, and birth emphasize apana vayu, the downward-moving energy we count on to move the baby down and out of the womb, as well as to regulate urination and defecation and keep us grounded. Our prenatal yoga practice consisted of squats, hip openers, and poses that created space between the ribcage and the pubic bone to give the baby room to grow and then descend. According to ayurvedic practitioner Niika Quistgard, this increased apana vayu must now recede to restore the integrity of the pelvic muscles and organs and to readjust the excess space that exists where the baby had taken up residence.

Western physical therapists, like Jessica McKinny, who directs the Center for Pelvic and Women's Health in Boston, have a different way of describing this early postpartum healing. Jessica says that excess weight and downward pressure can put a lot of strain on the pelvic floor muscles, which lengthen significantly, and can even tear during pregnancy. In the final three months, the superficial abdominal muscles (recti abdomini or "six-pack" muscles) move wider apart to accommodate an ever-expanding belly, making it even harder to breathe fully. This inability to breathe properly further compromises these muscles and causes a disconnect between the pelvic floor, diaphragm, and transverse abdominals—the innermost muscles that wrap around your middle and are partially responsible for a flatter belly. Postnatal posture plays a part as well. After all, your breasts are heavier now and you're nursing and holding your baby, all of which contribute to your shoulders collapsing forward. If you don't address this disconnect—and heal the recti abdomini split—before beginning a more physical practice, you run the risk of pelvic floor problems, including incontinence, organ prolapse, uterine pain, and constipation that can linger for years. Not to mention a poochy belly that never recedes no matter how many crunches you do.

GETTING OFF TO A SLOW START

Strengthening the diaphragm-pelvic floor connection is the first order of business, and you can start that as soon as you'd like after giving birth. You begin gently, of course, by connecting to the breath using Belly Breathing, Ujjayi Pranayama (Victorious Breath), and Nadi Shodhana (Alternate Nostril Breathing). Lying in a restorative pose such as Savasana (Corpse Pose) or Supta Virasana (Reclining Hero Pose), with plenty of support, provides a comfortable setting in which to experience that synergic connection and also to lightly engage and release your pelvic floor muscles. Practicing pranayama in a restorative pose or while nursing or rocking your baby, or even when you're lying down will also give you the opportunity to notice any places in your body that need your attention and then bathe them with healing breath.

Modified Nadi Shodhana (Alternate Nostril Breathing)

You can add this version of Nadi Shodhana to your pranayama practice anytime and anywhere; you don't even have to use your fingers to open or block your nostrils. Simply inhale up the left side of your torso into your left nostril and all the way to the top of your head; gently pause; and exhale out your right nostril, all the way down your right side, softening and nourishing your belly and reproductive organs. Pause after the exhalation. Next, slowly begin to inhale up your right side and pause before exhaling all the way out your left nostril. Do this for several rounds—5 to 7 minutes, if that works for you—and end on an exhalation on your left-hand side. This practice will help balance your nervous system, engage your pelvic floor, and give you a deeply relaxing and gently energizing experience.

STARTING FROM THE BOTTOM

Begin your practice by addressing the muscles, joints, ligaments and bones in the pelvis that worked extra hard all through your pregnancy, labor, and birth. Think of your pelvic floor as a hammock that holds everything up "down there." That hammock was pushed against and stretched open during labor and birthing. And no matter how you gave birth—vaginally or by cesarean—it was pummeled by the extra weight of the baby and its placenta and loosened by hormonal activity. It's now begun to sag and weaken and maybe even tear in places. A misaligned and destabilized pelvis might not cause you any immediate problems, but it could down the line, so it's important that you tone, stabilize, and realign your pelvis and pelvic floor muscles *before* moving on to abdominal work, vinyasa flows, or even standing or balancing poses. As B.K.S. Iyengar wrote in *Light on Life*, you need a firm foundation, a stable ground from which to move. So it makes a lot of sense physiologically and emotionally to begin reconnecting with—and strengthening—your roots.

Once you feel adept at contracting your pelvic floor muscles without gripping anywhere, you can move on to access your transverse abdominals (TAs), the muscles you can feel between your hip points. Dustienne Miller, a certified physical therapist and Kripalu yoga teacher, says that women usually have an easier time doing all this if gravity is eliminated. So begin your reentry journey on your back, exploring the connection between the pelvic floor and the TA muscles. Once you've nailed that, you can start activating the same muscles in standing postures, too.

DUSTIENNE'S GRAVITY-ELIMINATING FLOW PRACTICE

DUSTIENNE MILLER

In the following sequence, Dustienne encourages you to begin by practicing Belly Breathing and then do the poses lying on your back with your knees bent. If you're more comfortable, you can do any of these pelvic floor poses in Viparita Karani (Legs-Up-the-Wall Pose). Using Ujjayi Pranayama (Victorious Breath) throughout Dustienne's practice may help you move your breath into any tight or stuck places in your body.

Belly Breathing

Lie down with your feet on the floor and your knees in line with your hips. Place your hands on your abdomen, just under your belly button, in *yoni mudra* (a triangle shape with your index fingers at your pubic bone). Spend a few minutes inhaling and exhaling from your belly. Feel your sacrum heavy on the floor. As you inhale, feel your pelvic floor muscles widening out and down; as you exhale, notice them moving in and up.

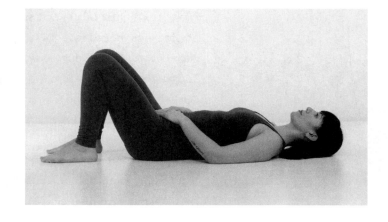

   Now, see if you can imagine inhaling and exhaling from the right side of your body. Focusing on your right sitting bone, expand out and down on the inhalation; gather and move in on the exhalation. Now try the left side.

The Elevator Lift

Imagine your pelvic floor as an elevator. As you inhale, without moving your torso, imagine the elevator gliding down to the first floor; as you exhale and actively pull the muscles up and in, it rises to the second floor. Inhale back to the first floor and on your next exhalation, move the muscles up to the third floor and inhale them back down.

BENEFITS: This exercise gently engages your pelvic floor muscles and begins to establish the connection between those muscles and your diaphragm in a relaxing supine position.

Pelvic Clocks

Lying in the same position, imagine you are on top of a clock face. Keeping your knees very still, tip your sacrum forward so it points to 12 o'clock and then flatten your lower back to move to 6 o'clock. Go back and forth several times between the two positions; return to a neutral position. Now move your sacrum from 3 o'clock to 9 o'clock several times. See how small you can make the movements; keep your knees still and only move your sacrum. Now starting at 12 o'clock, move your sacrum around the whole clock, focusing on your pelvis and sacrum. If you find that one part of the circle feels tighter or less accessible, stay there for a few breaths and notice any feelings that surface. When you get back to 12 o'clock, reverse the circle. Finally, move your sacrum on a diagonal from 11 o'clock to 5 o'clock and then from 1 o'clock to 7 o'clock. These movements are trickier and subtler than they sound, so just do what you can.

Hip Circles

Bring your right knee in toward your chest. With your right hand on the top of your kneecap and draw hip circles, moving one way for several breaths and then reversing the direction. Notice any restriction in your hip joint or in the muscle tissue around your hips and pelvis. Keep the sacrum nice and heavy on the floor. Release the right leg to the floor and change sides.

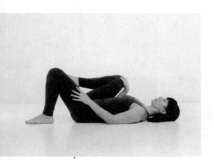
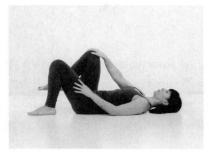
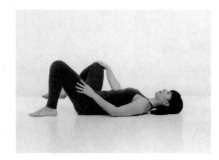

THE TRANSVERSE ABDOMINALS

Once you feel comfortable engaging and releasing your pelvic floor—and you can do so without pain—move your attention up to the transverse abdominal muscles and begin to gently engage them.

ISOMETRIC CONTRACTIONS

The transverse abdominals, the vital link between the diaphragm and the pelvic floor, are located between your two hip points (technically, the anterior superior iliac spine, or ASIS, bones). Continue to lie on your back with your feet on the floor and place your fingertips onto your hip points. Inhale. Then you exhale, imagine that a magnet is drawing these points together. This will produce a gentle contraction in your TA muscles. Repeat this awareness exercise 10 times.

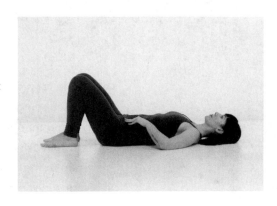

If you'd like to go deeper, keep your fingers on your hip points. Inhale. Then as you exhale, lift your right foot a few inches off the floor. On your next inhale, bring it down, and lift your left foot. The lifts should be small and your hip points should stay even. Repeat this exercise 8 to 10 times.

CAUTION: If you feel any straining, if your abdominals are pushing outward, if your hip points don't stay in the same plane, or if your back arches off the floor, you're doing too much. Back off a little until the strain is alleviated.

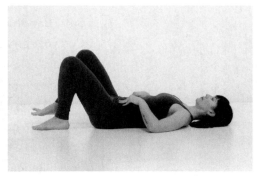

The Transverse Abdominal–Pelvic Floor Connection

Continue to lie on your back, returning your attention to your pelvic floor muscles. As you inhale, your belly expands up towards the ceiling and your pelvic floor muscles lengthen out and release down. As you exhale, your belly softly falls back towards your spine and your pelvic floor muscles lift and engage slightly. Do this awareness exercise 10 times.

If you feel a consistent engagement and release, practice coordinating your breath with the contraction of your pelvic floor and TA muscles together. Inhale for a count of 2, and feel your belly and pelvic floor muscles expand.

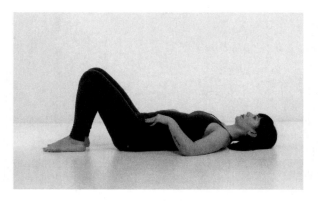
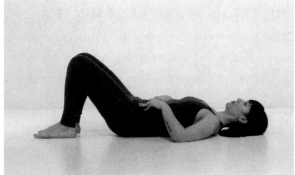

Exhale for a count of 2, gathering and lifting your pelvic floor muscles and scooping your lower belly in toward your spine. Increase the counts to 4 and then 6, if possible.

CAUTION: Once again, if your belly pooches out during the contraction, return to the first pelvic floor exercise. Visualize gathering the muscles and organs together and lifting them up and in.

Setu Bandha Sarvangasana (Bridge Pose)

Curl your pelvis under and lift your spine, one vertebra at a time, then let it down slowly, as though your vertebrae were a string of pearls. Place a block between your knees, if you wish, which will engage your inner thighs a bit more. Then, inhale to release your pelvic floor muscles and on your next exhalation, gather your pelvic floor and TA muscles up and in, and bridge up. Stay in a high bridge and pulse a little higher 5 times. Slowly roll back down. Repeat 3 times.

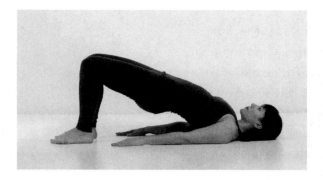

ALTERNATIVE

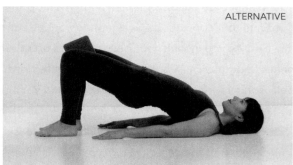

DUSTIENNE'S STANDING SEQUENCE

Once you feel comfortable engaging and releasing your pelvic floor muscles in a prone position, you can begin to explore that connection while standing. As always, do only as much as you feel capable of today and feel free to stay longer in each pose (or come out sooner).

Bird Dog Pose

Come onto your hands and knees. Soften your throat, jaw and face. Inhale, and as you exhale, lift and extend your right arm forward, holding this position for 3 to 5 breaths. Inhale as you release your right arm back down. Repeat with your left arm. With both hands on the floor, exhale as you extend and lift your left leg behind you, holding this position for 3 to 5 breaths and then as you inhale, release your foot to the floor. Repeat with your right leg.

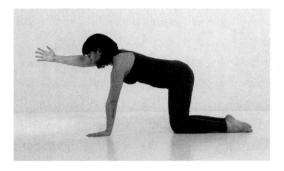
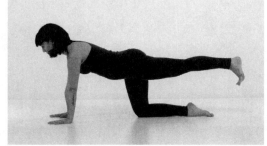

If you feel strong enough, inhale to prepare and then exhale to extend and lift your right arm and left leg together. Hold this position for 3 to 5 breaths and return to your hands and knees. Repeat with your left leg and right arm. See if you can feel a connection from your pelvic floor all the way to the crown of your head. Repeat 3 times each side.

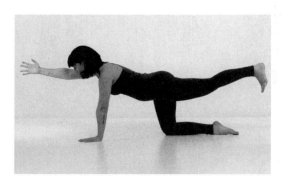

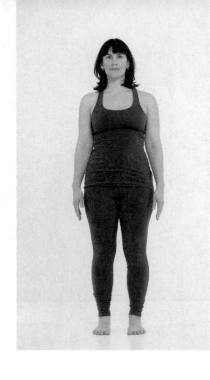

Tadasana (Mountain Pose)

Spend some time in Tadasana noticing your posture and placing your attention on your feet. Is there more weight in your heels than in your toes? Rock forward a little until your weight feels evenly distributed. Feel your feet move firmly into the ground; they are your foundation. Roll your shoulders back and allow them to gently descend down your back. Inhale up through your belly, ribcage, and collarbone; pause; exhale completely. Inhale and release your pelvic floor muscles; exhale and engage them gently. Do this 4 times.

Once you feel confident that you can contract and release your TA and pelvic floor muscles without straining, you can begin to access those muscles in standing poses. Add any of the following poses to the preceding sequence, or practice them on their own.

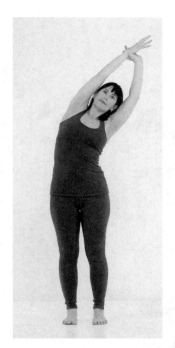 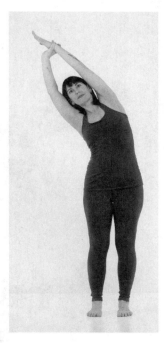

Parsva Urdhva Hastasana (Side-Bending Upward Salute)

Standing in Tadasana (Mountain Pose), inhale your arms overhead, extending through the sides of your body as you press down into your feet. Inhale as you clasp your right wrist and exhale as you lean to your left. Extend the breath into the right side of your body, keeping the weight even in both feet. Breathe here for 5 breaths; inhale to come up. Clasp your left wrist and exhale over to the right side, elongating your left side for 5 breaths. Slowly return to Urdhva Hastasana and then fold your hands at your heart in Tadasana.

Utkatasana (Chair Pose)

Place your hands on your hips, inhale and lower yourself into Utkatasana. On your next exhalation, gather and contract your pelvic floor muscles, and lift up to standing. Hold the contraction for 5 seconds. Repeat several times, if you wish.

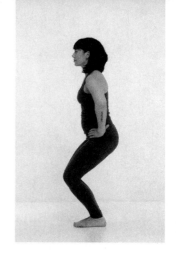

Virabhadrasana I (Warrior I) variation

If you feel strong enough, move into a high lunge—Virabhadrasana I with your back heel lifted. Inhale and bend your back knee. Exhale to gather and engage your pelvic floor muscles and straighten your back leg. Repeat this movement 4 times, then reverse legs and repeat. Keep your hands on your hips, or extend your arms out to the sides and overhead.

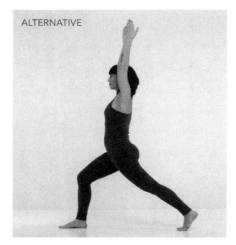

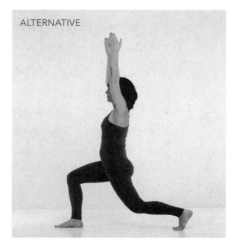

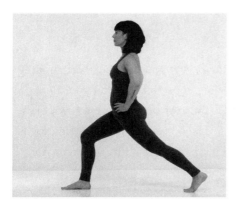

ALTERNATIVE

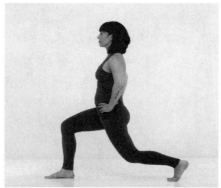

ALTERNATIVE

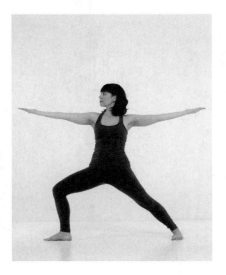

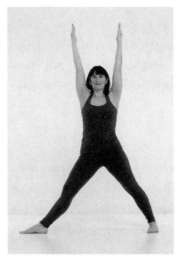

Virabhadrasana II (Warrior II) variation

From Virabhadrasana I move into Virabhadrasana II, with your arms out to the sides, palms facing up. On an inhalation, bend your front knee. As you exhale, gather and lift your pelvic floor muscles while straightening your legs and reaching your arms overhead. Do this movement a few times, then reverse legs and repeat.

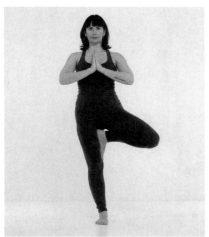

Vrksasana (Tree Pose)

Begin in Tadasana (Mountain Pose) with your feet hip-width apart. Inhale to release your pelvic floor muscles. And on your next exhalation, gather and lift those muscles up as you press your left foot into your right inner thigh (as high up as you feel comfortable). Bring your hands to your heart in prayer position and remain in the pose for 5 breaths, if possible.

Baddha Konasana (Bound Angle Pose)

Sit up tall on a folded blanket, with the soles of your feet together. If you feel tired, sit with your back against a wall. Relax your jaw, soften your tongue, and allow your knees to descend toward the mat. Stay in this position as long as you are comfortable, practicing your Belly Breathing and releasing your inner thighs and pelvic floor muscles.

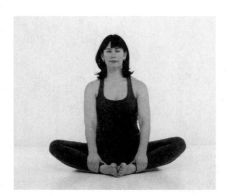

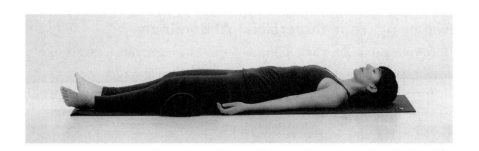

Savasana (Corpse Pose)

Lie down in Savasana for 10 minutes, or as long as you like, paying particular attention to the your breath, softening your belly, your hip flexors, and your groin and allowing your sacrum to feel heavy on the mat.

Navigating the Pelvic Floor Muscles

It may be hard to figure out how to contract your pelvic floor muscles correctly. Depending on your comfort level, you can try any of the following:

- Insert your finger into your vaginal opening and squeeze gently. You should feel the muscles lifting up and in, gripping your finger. You should not feel a pushing out or a bulging sensation.
- With a mirror, take a look at your nether regions. When you contract your pelvic floor muscles, you may see your anus puckering a little and your clitoris "nodding."
- When you contract your pelvic floor muscles, visualize your sitting bones moving toward each other. Imagine lifting up a pearl with your labia.
- When you contract your transverse abdominals, visualize your hip points moving toward each other.
- When you contract your pelvic floor and transverse abdominal muscles, imagine you are zipping up a pair of low-rise jeans.
- If you start bleeding, notice abnormal vaginal discharge, or feel pain, numbness, burning, or tingling, stop your practice and talk with your doctor. Stop also if your intuition tells you you've done too much, too quickly.

Repairing Your Superficial Abdominals

Once your pelvic floor and TA muscles feel stronger and are working in concert with your diaphragm, you can slowly begin to knit your outermost abdominal muscles back together again. These are the six-pack muscles most women are so eager to reclaim. The recti abdomini are two long, flat muscles that run parallel to each another along the front of the body, separated at the midline and held together by connective tissue called linea alba. These abdominals stretch and pull apart during pregnancy to accommodate your growing uterus. After you give birth, they move back towards each other, but don't always come back together in the same way, resulting in what is called a diastasis, or separation. If the diastasis isn't treated or addressed, it may result in incontinence; lower back pain; weakened pelvic floor muscles; and what women decry as their "mommy belly," the discouraging pooch that seems to linger long after baby is born.

Unfortunately, all the sit-ups and crunches they do in hopes of strengthening their core only make things worse. Jeanie Manchester, a

How to Check for Diastasis

1. Look at your belly button first. If you now have an "outie" that used to be an "innie," or if your belly button kind of droops or sags, your connective tissue hasn't fully drawn the recti abdomini back together.
2. You can feel a diastasis gap in three different places. Lie down with your knees bent and your feet flat on the floor. First, place one hand on your abdomen. Press your fingers into your belly button and slowly lift your head, just until you feel your abdominal muscles engaging, and see if you can feel a gap between the two sides of the muscle. The gap may be the width of one finger or several. Second, move your fingers to about three inches above your belly button and do the same test. Third, check the area three inches below your belly button.

strong Boulder, Colorado–based vinyasa teacher, learned the hard way with her second child. She went back to her normal Ashtanga practice before her diastasis healed. "I began to do backbends too soon," she says, ending up with severe back pain. Although she eased up and worked on strengthening her pelvic floor, it's taken her 16 years of pranayama, Mula Bandha (Root Lock), and conscious pelvic floor work to heal.

Jessica McKinny, the Boston-area physical therapist and pelvic floor expert, says most women have some degree of diastasis immediately after they give birth because the separation was Nature's way of creating more room for the baby to grow. The majority of these splits resolve themselves, but at least 25 percent are still present eight weeks postpartum. Take the time to resolve your diastasis, if you have one, because although you may not experience any immediate ill effects, you could end up having problems five, ten, or even twenty years down the road (especially during hormonally charged menopause).

Luckily, the same pranayama practices that you do to consciously breathe into your belly will help knit things back together. The more you're able to reconnect your pelvic floor and the TA muscles, which are neurologically hardwired to work together, the more efficiently and quickly you'll be able to repair your superficial abdominals.

WHAT NOT TO DO

Resist the urge to do poses that engage the recti abdomini, including crunches, Paripurna Navasana (Boat Pose), or Ardha Navasana (Half Boat Pose). Doing any kind of "sit-up" poses will make a split worse rather than better, because they put outward pressure on the muscle. If your diastasis is pronounced, De West says to avoid poses that compromise your posture or poses that "put the weight of your organs on your abdominal split" like Adho Mukha Svanasana (Downward-Facing Dog Pose). Do not do arm balances or closed twists like Marichyasana III (Marichi's Pose) either.

WHAT TO FOCUS ON

If you do have a fairly pronounced diastasis, do the Pelvic Rocks here, as well as Dustienne's Gravity-Eliminating Flow Practice on page 193, to simultaneously engage your transverse abdominals, which are partially responsible for a flatter belly, and your pelvic floor muscles. Stay connected to your breath. Once you establish that connection, focus on standing poses that encourage good posture and proper alignment of your pelvis. These poses will help strengthen your TA muscles, engage your pelvic floor muscles, and heal your recti abdomini.

Pelvic Rocks

Lie on your back, with your feet flat on the floor, hip-width apart. Inhale completely; as you exhale, tuck your belly button in toward your spine and lift the tip of your tailbone slightly. Inhale as you release your tailbone down and gently arch your back. Rock your pelvis back and forth several times—work up to 20 reps—gently engaging your deeper abdominals.

CAUTION: This is a subtle exercise. You should feel your lower abdominals engage, but you shouldn't feel any movement elsewhere in your body, including your knees. Keep your throat, jaw, neck, and chest relaxed.

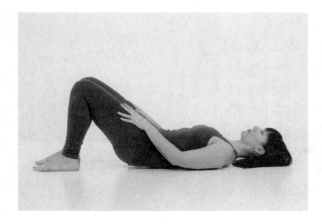 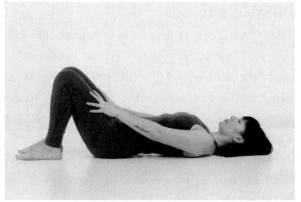

HOW TO IMPROVE YOUR POSTURE

Besides practices that will help heal the pelvic floor and abdominal muscles and rebalance the nervous system, most women crave poses that will release their shoulders, neck, and upper back, all of which become increasingly scrunched from holding and nursing. Not only do the following poses counter the physical challenges of being a new mom, but they also make you feel better: Tadasana (Mountain Pose), Vrksasana (Tree Pose), Adho Mukha Svanasana (Downward-Facing Dog), Virabhradasana I and II (Warrior Poses) and Parsva Urdhva Hastasana (Side-Bending Upward Salute).

Reclaiming Your Practice as a New Yoga Mama

The yoga world has a lot to offer women during pregnancy and the early postpartum months—plenty of prenatal and "Baby & Me" classes and suggestions for getting back into shape. But once their kids are moving more and sleeping less, many women feel a little lost and wonder if they'll ever be able to get their yoga practice back.

It helps to remember that yoga begins wherever you are. No doubt that's an adage you've heard a thousand times, but it's especially true for the infant-into-toddler years. If this is your second or third child, you may feel the separation from your yoga practice more acutely, especially if your children are close in age. You probably need your practice more than ever, yet the time, energy, and motivation may not be there. Instead of giving up, take time to decide what you need most from yoga right now, especially if you're still struggling to find a way to care for yourself. Do you need a time-out to hide away and recharge? Does your body crave movement or deep relaxation? Can you practice with your baby or is that too distracting?

Laura Erdman-Luntz, a Minnesota yoga teacher, couldn't wait to get back to yoga. Pre-baby, her practice meant pranayama, meditation twice a day, and a full asana session. Once she brought her baby home, she quickly realized that routine was not going to happen again anytime soon. She had to let go of what she did before and be fine with ten deep breaths in the morning before getting out of bed, a two-minute Tree Pose while she brushed her teeth, and a stay-awhile Cobra Pose, low enough to the ground that she could talk and coo to her baby. Some days her practice consisted of a single pose or a few minutes of pranayama; other days, she had a little more time and energy.

As new mothers, we often feel conflicted. We pour all the love and energy and time we have into our babies and somehow forget about channeling some of it into caring for ourselves. Kate Hanley, whose practice suggestions show up later in this chapter, has two small children to care for. She convinced herself that everything would work more smoothly if she just put whatever time she had for yoga into her "duties" as a mom.

Seven Opportunities to Build Meditation into Your Day

Yoga doesn't always mean asana or even pranayama. A meditation practice can sometimes be easier to fold into your day than time on your mat. Even a few moments of quiet time, as Kate Hanley's suggestions here demonstrate, can refresh you and help you recommit to caring for yourself and your baby:

- Meditate while nursing.
- Do a walking meditation when you are waiting for your child to fall asleep.
- Practice conscious breathing while you cook or clean.
- Do a listening meditation. Focus as much of your attention as you can spare on what you can hear, not distinguishing between sounds but registering each one as it passes while you commute, have your morning coffee on the porch, or walk the dog.
- When you go out for a walk, sit down in a lovely spot and meditate for a brief but deeply effective five minutes before you return home.
- When your child falls asleep in the car, sit and meditate for five minutes or so before you get the car seat out or wake her up.
- Meditate for three minutes before you get out of bed in the morning.

"It became so easy to put the kids first and me last," she told me. But the physical and emotional demands—no sleep, lots of sitting (for rocking and nursing), poor posture from holding a baby on one side of her body as she attempted to cook—soon took their toll. When she finally decided she'd meditate whenever she nursed her infant son to sleep, she almost immediately felt her whole body and mind settle down. From there, she says, "I started making my nightly sweeping (since we produced a mountain of crumbs and crushed Crayons in those days) an exercise in mindfulness. I let myself feel the weight of the broom in my hands, the rhythm of my body as it slowly moved around the room, the sound of the bristles swishing against the floor." Those two activities became her basic practice, and she slowly began to add other mindful practices whenever she could.

Redefining Your Practice

The last thing you want is to make yoga one more item on a long "must-do" list. You have enough obligations already. Yoga should become a companion, a way of energizing, nourishing, and supporting yourself no matter where you are in your postnatal journey. Sometimes it's enough to draw on the cumulative kinesthetic effects of your years of yoga, even if you aren't ready to get back on your mat. Claudia Cummins, writer and yogini, didn't practice any postures for quite a while after giving birth: "Although I missed my devoted practices, I began to see that, for me, new motherhood didn't seem like the right season for a lot of yoga." That said, Claudia thinks her years of practice beforehand paid off. "I felt like my practice had packed me full of some clean and long-lasting yoga fuel that was still pumping through my veins," she says. "And I believe that all that past yoga helped my body bounce back on its own fairly quickly."

Reuniting with tapas, svadhyaya, and ishvara pranidhana—discipline, self-reflection, and surrender—can help you figure out what you need right now. You may even want to turn things upside down and begin with surrender! In other words, surrender any preconceived notion of what yoga should look like and what you have to accomplish before you can really call it yoga. Then spend some moments in self-reflection (perhaps when you're nursing or taking a walk). What would serve you best? Would you feel more rejuvenated, calmer, and happier if you could hand off your little one to your partner or a good friend and take a postnatal class or do a 30-minute practice of your own? Or would you love a nap instead? Then engage your inner willpower (tapas) and determination to take time for yourself, reaching out to your partner and friends to help you make that happen.

Finding Time for Yoga

As Laura discovered, you sometimes need to get creative—a backbend over the kitchen counter to offset the effects of holding and nursing, a standing twist at the changing table to get the kinks out—in order to get any kind of practice in during your day. It might sound a little silly, but don't discount the little spaces between your obligations. They provide essential practice time, even for just a few moments. Kate came up with some mini sequences that she felt were lifesavers when she was a new mother. Choose the ones that work for you, and by all means, have some fun creating new ones.

CHANGING TABLE VINYASA

You've got to change diapers several times a day, so you may as well do a few poses while you're at it. It's fairly easy to pay attention to your baby and reduce tension in your shoulders, neck, and back at the same time. Practice a few poses once or twice, depending on how long your baby is content to stay on the table.

- Urdvha Hastasana (Upward Salute) is an opportunity to untangle your spine and give your organs a little more space so you can breathe and digest more fully. As you stack your shoulders over hips and your hips over your ankles, be careful not to lean into the side of the changing table. Raise your arms over your head, interlace your fingers, and turn your palms to the ceiling. Encourage your shoulder blades to move down, away from your ears, as you lift your ribcage up and off your pelvic floor. Reach down through your feet and up through your palms to come to your maximum height.

- Parsva Urdhva Hastasana (Side-Bending Upward Salute) will engage your oblique abdominals, which you may not have felt in a while, and move your breath up into your chest for an energy-booster. Just take hold of your right wrist, reach up tall, and bend to your left side. Inhale back up to center, switch hands, and exhale as you side bend to the right.

- Tadasana (Mountain Pose), the quintessential "fake-it-till-you-make-it" pose, can strengthen your legs, ground your energy, and elongate your spine. Placing your hands behind your back in reverse prayer position will spread your collarbones wider and counter the rounding you already feel in your upper spine from holding and nursing your baby. Since it moves your breath up into your chest, Tadasana done this way may help relieve the baby blues.

COFFEE-BREWING VINYASA

When your baby (hopefully) sleeps in the arms of your partner, put that time to good use. Use the kitchen counter to stretch and wake your body up naturally, while the coffee or tea finishes brewing.

- Ardha Adho Mukha Svanasana (Half Downward-Facing Dog Pose) can stretch out your whole back and release your hamstrings. Place your fingertips shoulder-width apart on the edge of counter. Walk your feet back as you hinge at the hips until your spine is fully extended and your feet are directly under your hips. Look at the floor so the back of your neck lengthens. Staying here for several breaths is a great way to align your spine and get the kinks out.
- Virabhadrasana III (Warrior III) follows organically from Ardha Adho Mukha Svanasana and lets you engage your deeper core muscles and check your balance. So, hold on to the counter's edge as you lift your back leg to hip height and rotate it inward, which will keep your knee and hipbone pointing down toward the floor and your hips level. And then repeat all this on the other side.
- Utthita Hasta Padangusthasana (Extended Hand-to-Toe Pose) is another way to strengthen and stretch your legs, engage your abs, and enliven your mood. Back up so you're about a leg's length from the counter, stretch out your right leg and place your right heel on the counter's edge. To get more space and breath into the sides of your body, reach your arms overhead and lift your ribs off your pelvis. If your hamstrings are crying out for attention, too, bend from your hips and reach out for your right calf or foot. Repeat on your left side. If your counter is too tall, find a lower table or press your foot against a cabinet at hip height.

SHOWER POWER VINYASA

At this point in your life, the shower may be the only place you truly get some alone time. It's not a bad place to hide out while the restorative power of water soothes and rejuvenates you.

....

- Ardha Adho Mukha Svanasana (Half Downward-Facing Dog Pose), with the water hitting your back just right, is a heavenly way to fire up your hamstrings, realign your spine, release your head and neck and be beholden to the restorative power of hot water to relieve any physical and emotional tension. Take several breaths and feel all the tension wash away.
- Tadasana (Mountain Pose) can provide a little mood-enhancing, back-bending magic in the shower. Stand facing the showerhead and interlace your hands behind you, straighten your arms and reach your knuckles toward the floor. Lengthen your spine so your upper back lifts up and back and your sternum faces the ceiling. Look at the ceiling or drop your head back, whichever feels better, and let the water fall on your upper chest and throat. Staying here for several breaths increases circulation to and nourishes your thyroid, which helps regulate metabolism and energy levels.
- Head Hanging Tadasana may be just what the doctor ordered to release muscular tension in the back of your neck. This time face away from the showerhead and allow your arms to dangle by your sides. Lift your ribs off your hips as you imagine your collarbones releasing away from each other. Drop your head toward your chest and let the water hit the back of your neck.

Take Savasana Breaks

Even though sleep may elude you, lying in Savasana (Corpse Pose) can help restore your body and keep your energy and spirits up. Rest for 10 to 15 minutes at a time, as often as you can sneak it into your routine. Here are some suggestions:

- Right after you put your child down to sleep. Although people always tell mothers to sleep when their babies and toddlers sleep, that's not always possible, especially if your little one isn't much of a sleeper. So if you can't sleep, do Savasana for 10 minutes before you tackle anything else.
- Right after the sitter or your partner takes the kids outside or to the park. Again, practice first, and everything you do after will be easier and more gratifying.
- While the coffee brews. On those days when you're physically exhausted, allow yourself to rest in Savasana on the living room floor while you wait for that first cup of coffee or your afternoon tea.

Nursing Pranayama and Meditation

Meditating while nursing her baby to sleep is what led Kate back toward a regular body-mind practice, helped her be more present (and pleasant), and able to savor closeness with her son. She also felt that her quiet energy helped him drift off to sleep. The technique doesn't matter so much as your commitment to starting again whenever you notice your attention has wandered—as it will, particularly on days tinged with sleeplessness-induced brain fog. Kate shares three examples of simple mindfulness exercises you can do while you're nursing or even while you're standing outside your little one's room, making sure he's truly asleep.

FOCUS ON YOUR EXHALATIONS

Instead of counting your inhalations and exhalations, bring your awareness to each exhalation, lightly touching in with your mind. When your attention wanders away from the present moment, simply notice and come back to the exhalation. This particular meditation helps you rein in straying thoughts and reminds you that keeping things simple can still be incredibly powerful.

INHALE PEACE, EXHALE STRESS

Imagine a color that symbolizes relaxation to you (mine is a Mediterranean blue). Then call to mind a color that represents toxic stress, such as a crimson red or a murky brown. As you inhale, imagine your peaceful color filling your every cell; as you exhale, imagine every iota of stress (encapsulated in the toxic color) being drained from your body and expelled out into the air. This practice gives you a visual focus for those moments when a more traditional meditation feels too challenging or uninspiring.

INHALE, EXHALE, PAUSE

Rest your attention on your belly, becoming aware of the rise and fall of the breath. Inhale three, four, or five counts (whatever feels like a complete breath without straining), pause, and exhale the same number of counts (or slightly longer). Now bring your awareness to and begin to lengthen the pause between your exhalation and your next inhalation. During that pause, let go of all effort: soften and release your shoulders, lower jaw, lips, and eyes. This pranayama practice allows you to slow down, trusting in the quiet space that happens naturally between each breath. It also relieves anxious thoughts, releases tension, and promotes relaxation—all good ways to encourage your milk to let down.

Tools for Sleep

Of all the tolls motherhood exacts on your body, exhaustion is probably the worst. It affects everything—your thinking process, your food choices, your mood. Try one of these two simple and fundamental practices to get the rest that will restore you.

EXTENDED EXHALATION BREATHING

Lying on your back, begin by inhaling and exhaling to a count of three or four each. Once you've established an even rhythm and feel your nervous system quiet down and your body sink into the mattress, lengthen your exhalations. Inhale for a count of three and exhale for six. Play with the count, but try to make your exhalations twice as long as your inhalations. As you exhale, visualize your body letting go of any tension, and picture your mind releasing all extraneous thoughts or difficult emotions.

SIMPLE ACUPRESSURE

Lie on your back with one palm resting on your heart and the other on your solar plexus. Stay here a few minutes until you start to feel drowsy, then move your top hand to your lower belly, just below your navel. The meridian (energy pathway) that runs down the front of your torso is the Conception Vessel, and it contains your most primal energy. Resting your hands on it lightly helps soothe this energy and your spirit, allowing you to release into sleep.

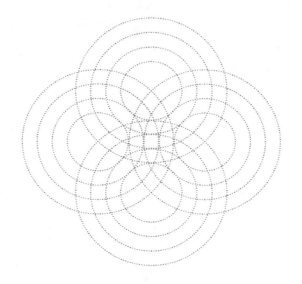

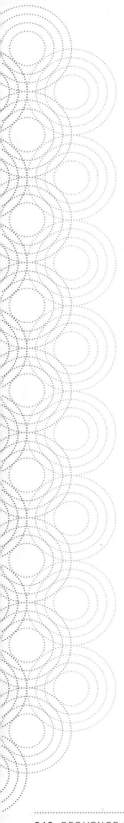

SEQUENCE GUIDE

Here's a quick and easy way to access the sequences you need whenever you need them.

My Morning Sickness Sequence (page 16)

Sukhasana (Easy Seated Pose) with Arm Movements

Vajrasana Surya Namaskar (Thunderbolt Sun Salutation)

Tadasana (Mountain Pose)

Ardha Surya Namaskar (Mini Sun Salutation)

Vrksasana (Tree Pose)

Ardha Chandrasana (Half-Moon Pose)

Sukhasana (Easy Seated Pose)

Balasana (Child's Pose)

Supta Virasana (Reclining Hero Pose)

Savasana (Corpse Pose)

Melissa's Fatigue Sequence (page 22)

Balasana (Child's Pose)

Uttana Shishosana (Extended Puppy Pose)

Adho Mukha Svanasana (Downward-Facing Dog Pose)

Virabhadrasana II (Warrior II Pose)

Utthita Trikonasana (Extended Triangle Pose)

Welcoming and Accepting: Your First Trimester Practice (page 27)

Shoulder Rolls

Sukhasana (Easy Seated Pose) Circles

Marjaryasana to Bitilasana in Sukhasana (Cat/Cow Pose), Seated Variation

Tadasana (Mountain Pose) with Circle Variations

Surya Namaskar (Sun Salutation)

    Tadasana (Mountain Pose)

    Urdhva Hastasana (Upward Salute)

    Uttanasana (Standing Forward Bend)

Ardha Uttanasana (Half Standing Forward Bend)

Phalakasana (Plank Pose)

Bhujangasana (Cobra Pose) or Urdhva Mukha Svanasana
(Upward-Facing Dog Pose)

Adho Mukha Svanasana (Downward-Facing Dog Pose)

Uttanasana (Standing Forward Bend)

Urdhva Hastasana (Upward Salute)

Tadasana (Mountain Pose)

Parsva Utkata Konasana (Side-Stretching Goddess Pose)

Virabhadrasana II (Warrior II Pose)

Utthita Parsvakonasana (Extended Side-Angle Pose)

Virabhadrasana II (Warrior II Pose)

Viparita Virabhadrasana (Reverse Warrior Pose)

Ardha Chandrasana (Half-Moon Pose)

Utthita Trikonasana (Extended Triangle Pose)

Parsvottansana (Intense Side Stretch)

Uttanasana (Standing Forward Bend)

Adho Mukha Svanasana (Downward-Facing Dog Pose)

Malasana (Garland Pose)

Baddha Konasana (Bound Angle Pose)

Paschimottanasana (Seated Forward Bend)

Savasana (Corpse Pose)

Melissa's Sequence for Indigestion (page 52)

Anjaneyasana (Low Lunge)

Supta Baddha Konasana (Reclining Bound Angle Pose)

Balasana (Child's Pose)

Side-Lying Savasana (Corpse Pose)

Sukhasana (Easy Seated Pose) Variation

Melissa's Sequence for Hip and Pelvic Pain (page 55)

Agni Stambhasana (Fire Log Pose)

Malasana (Garland Pose)

Eka Pada Rajakapotasana (Pigeon Pose)

Rooting Down and Looking Within: Your Second Trimester Practice (page 63)

Sukhasana (Easy Seated Pose) variations

    Marjaryasana to Bitilasana (Cat/Cow Cycle) Variation

    Spinal circles

Calf Stretch

Tail Wag

Uttana Shishosana (Extended Puppy Pose)

Adho Mukha Svanasana (Downward-Facing Dog Pose)

    Adho Mukha Svanasana (Downward-Facing Dog Pose) to Phalakasana (Plank Pose) to Adho Mukha Svanasana

    Chaturanga Dandasana (Four-Legged Staff Pose)

    Urdhva Mukha Svanasana (Upward-Facing Dog Pose)

    Adho Mukha Svanasana (Downward-Facing Dog Pose)

Uttanasana (Standing Forward Bend)

Virabhadrasana II (Warrior II Pose) Variation

Tadasana (Mountain Pose)

Virabhadrasana II (Warrior II) Variation

Utthita Trikonasana (Extended Triangle Pose)

Virabhadrasana II to Utthita Parsvakonasana (Warrior II Pose to Extended Side-Angle Pose)

Utkata Konasana (Goddess Pose)

Prasarita Padottanasana (Wide-Legged Standing Forward Bend)

Parivritta Prasarita Padottanasana (Revolved Wide-Legged Standing Forward Bend)

Virabhadrasana I (Warrior I)

Uttanasana (Standing Forward Bend)

One-Legged Hip Circles

Adho Mukha Svanasana (Downward-Facing Dog Pose)

Malasana (Garland Pose)

Janu Sirsasana (Head-on-Knee Pose)

Sukhasana (Easy Seated Pose) with Twist

Baddha Konasana (Bound Angle Pose)

Upavistha Konasana (Wide-Angle Seated Pose)

Side-Lying Savasana (Corpse Pose)
Seated Meditation

Asanas for the Pelvic Floor (page 90)
Virasana (Hero Pose)
Polar Bear Pose
Pelvic Tilts
Hip Circles
Figure Eights
Wave Squats

Listening and Releasing: Your Third Trimester Practice (page 122)
Seated Warm-ups
Marjaryasana to Bitilasana (Cat/Cow Cycle) with Variations
Pelvic Circles
Thread the Needle
Adho Mukha Svanasana (Downward-Facing Dog Pose)
Uttanasana (Standing Forward Bend)
Tadasana (Mountain Pose)
Pelvic Figure Eights
Surya Namaskar (Sun Salutation)
   Tadasana (Mountain Pose)
   Urdhva Hastasana (Upward Salute)
   Parsva Urdhva Hastasana (Sidebending Upward Salute)
   Urdhva Hastasana (Upward Salute)
   Uttanasana (Standing Forward Bend)
   Ardha Uttanasana (Half Standing Forward Bend)
   High Lunge
   Adho Muhka Svanasana (Downward-Facing Dog Pose)
   Phalakasana (Plank Pose)
   Ustrasana (Camel Pose)
   Adho Mukha Svanasana (Downward-Facing Dog Pose)
   High Lunge

Anjaneyasana (Low Lunge)

Uttanasana (Standing Forward Bend)

Tadasana (Mountain Pose)

Virabhadrasana II (Warrior II Pose)

Utthita Trikonasana (Extended Triangle Salute)

Tadasana (Mountain Pose)

Ardha Chandrasana (Half-Moon Pose)

Prasarita Padottanasana (Wide-Legged Standing Forward Bend)

Utkatasana (Chair Pose)

Sacrum Massage

Supta Baddha Konasana (Reclining Bound Angle Pose)

Side-Lying Savasana (Corpse Pose)

Positioning Baby Poses (pages 153, 167)

Shaking the Apples (Uttana Shoshosana)

Humming Dolphin

Connecting and Supporting: Partner Yoga (page 160)

SUN SALUTATION DUETS

Tadasana (Mountain Pose)

Ardha Malasana (Half Garland Pose)

Urdhva Hastasana (Upward Salute)

Ardha Uttanasana (Half Standing Forward Bend)

Uttanasana (Standing Forward Bend)

Malasana (Garland Pose)

Urdhva Hastasana (Upward Salute)

Tadasana (Mountain Pose)

PARTNER SQUATTING VINYASA

Malasana (Garland Pose)

Malasana to Bitilasana (Cat/Cow Cycle), asymmetrical variation

Pelvic Rocks

Balasana (Child's Pose)

Malasana (Garland Pose)

Flowing with the Breath: Sound and Movement for Birth (page 166)

Vajrasana Surya Namaskar (Kneeling Sun Salutation)

    Vajrasana (Thunderbolt Pose)

    Urdhva Hastasana (Upward Salute)

Humming Dolphin

Hissing Fish

Mama Salutes with Sound

    Tadasana (Mountain Pose)

    Urdhva Hastasana (Upward Salute)

    Uttanasana (Standing Forward Bend)

    Ardha Uttanasana (Half Standing Forward Bend)

    High Lunge

    Anjaneyasana (Low Lunge)

    Marjaryasana to Bitilasana (Cat/Cow Cycle)

    Anjaneyasana (Low Lunge)

    High Lunge

    Ardha Uttanasana (Half Forward Bend)

    Urdhva Hastasana (Upward Salute)

    Tadasana (Mountain Pose)

Virabhadrasana I Flow

    Tadasana (Mountain Pose)

    Virabhadrasana I (Warrior I Pose)

Seated Flow—Moaning

    Upavistha Konasana (Wide-Angle Seated Pose)

    Baddha Konasana (Bound Angle Pose)

    Upavistha Konasana (Wide-Angle Seated Pose)

    Sukhasana (Easy Seated Pose)

Dustienne's Gravity-Eliminating Flow (page 193)

Belly Breathing

The Elevator Lift

Pelvic Clocks

Hip Circles

ISOMETRIC CONTRACTIONS
Transverse Abdominal/Pelvic Floor Connection
Setu Bandha Sarvangasana (Bridge Pose)

Dustienne's Standing Sequence (page 197)
Bird Dog Pose
Tadasana (Mountain Pose)
Parsva Urdhva Hastasana (Side-Bending Upward Salute)
Utkatasana (Chair Pose)
Virabhadrasana I (Warrior I Pose) Variation
Virabhadrasana II (Warrior II Pose)
Vrksasana (Tree Pose)
Baddha Konasana (Bound Angle Pose)
Savasana (Corpse Pose)

RESOURCES

Pre- and Postnatal DVDs

(available on amazon.com unless otherwise indicated)

Breech Birth and Shoulder Dystocia with Ina May Gaskin (inamay.com)

Element: Prenatal & Postnatal Yoga with Elena Brower

Prenatal Yoga with Jane Austin (janeaustinyoga.com)

Your Pace Yoga: Relieving Pelvic Pain with Dustienne Miller

Your Pace Yoga: Optimizing Bladder Control with Dustienne Miller

Documentary Films

Birth Story: Ina May Gaskin and the Farm Midwives, a film by Sara Lamm and Mary Wigmore (produced by Kate Roughan and Zachary Mortensen)

Breastmilk, a film by Dana Ben-Ari (produced by Ricki Lake and Abby Epstein)

The Business of Being Born, a film by Dana Ben-Ari (produced by Ricki Lake and Abby Epstein)

The Face of Birth, a film by Kate Gorman (produced by Baby Banksia)

Online Resources

PRENATAL YOGA

Prenatalyogacenter.com

Yogaglo.com

Anytimeyoga.com

Mayoga.com

Janeaustinyoga.com

BIRTHING CHALLENGES

Inamay.com

Spinningbabies.com

MIDWIFERY AND DOULAS

Mana.org (Midwives Alliance of North America)

Dona.org (International organization for birth and postpartum doulas)

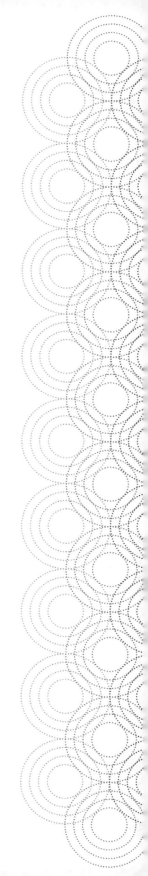

Supplemental Reading

Be Fruitful, by Victoria Maizes (Simon and Schuster)

Birthing from Within, by Pam England (Partera Press)

Birth Matters, by Ina May Gaskin and Ani DiFranco (Seven
Stories Press)

Bountiful, Beautiful, Blissful, by Gurmukh (St. Martin's Griffin)

Gentle Birth, Gentle Mothering, by Sarah Buckley, MD (Celestial Arts)

Ina May's Guide to Breastfeeding, by Ina May Gaskin (Bantam Press)

Ina May's Guide to Childbirth, by Ina May Gaskin (Bantam Press)

Pelvic Power, by Eric Franklin (Elysian Editions)

Preparing for a Gentle Birth: The Pelvis in Pregnancy,
by Blandine Calais-Germain (Healing Arts Press)

ABOUT THE CONTRIBUTING TEACHERS

Jane Austin

Passionate about yoga and the transformative power of motherhood, Jane works with pre- and postnatal mamas. As a mom herself, she has been a doula and childbirth educator since 1990. As founding director of Mama Tree, she trains yoga teachers, birth professionals, and others to teach pre- and postnatal yoga. You can find online classes and her DVD, *Prenatal Yoga with Jane Austin*, on janeaustinyoga.com.

Elena Brower

Mama, teacher, speaker, and coauthor of *Art of Attention*, Elena has taught yoga since 1999. Influenced by several traditions, she offers international yoga and meditation classes as a way to approach our world with reverence and gratitude. A masterful blend of artful alignment and attention cues for the body, mind, and heart, her classes are also available on yogaglo.com and elenabrower.com.

Sarah Buckley, MD

New Zealand–trained family physician Sarah Buckley is the author of *Gentle Birth, Gentle Mothering: A Doctor's Guide to Natural Childbirth and Gentle Early Parenting Choices*. Her ongoing interest in the hormones of labor and birth has culminated in her groundbreaking report *Hormonal Physiology of Childbearing*, published with Childbirth Connection, a program of the National Partnership for Women and Families. She encourages us to be fully informed in our decision-making; to listen to our hearts and our intuition; and to claim our rightful role as the real experts in our bodies and our children.

Kate Hanley

Kate Hanley is a life coach, yoga teacher, writer, and speaker. She is passionate about helping busy people find meaningful ways to slow

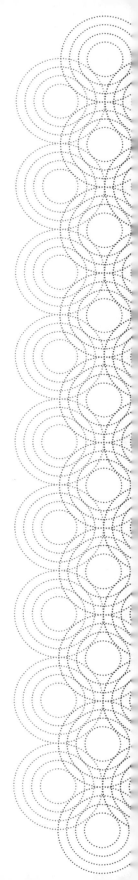

down and hear what's true for them. The author of *The Anywhere, Anytime Chill Guide* and coauthor of *The 28 Days Lighter Diet*, Kate brings the message that even short, nontraditional forms of practice can keep you sane, grounded, and happy. You can visit her at msmindbody.com.

Dustienne Miller

Dustienne is a yoga teacher and a board-certified women's clinical health specialist recognized through the American Board of Physical Therapy Specialties. Her DVDs—*Your Pace Yoga: Relieving Pelvic Pain* and *Your Pace Yoga: Optimizing Bladder Control*—have been adopted and endorsed by physical therapists, physicians, and other medical professionals. Look for more information at yourpaceyoga.com.

Stephanie Snyder

The creator of the *Yoga Journal* DVD, *Yoga for Strength and Toning*, Stephanie's commitment to breath, movement, happiness, and prayer make her one of America's most sought-after teachers. She is indebted to Sri Dharma Mittra for sharing with her the real heart of the practice. Her pre- and postnatal offerings can be found on yogaglo.com. You can also visit her at stephaniesnyder.com.

De West

De is an insightful, intuitive, and attentive teacher, who generously shares her love of yoga in a nonjudgmental, compassionate way. Precision, attention to breath, and a deep understanding of anatomy contribute to her ability to help her students connect with their innate intelligence. Her innovative Prenatal/Postpartum Yoga Teacher Intensive draws practitioners from across the United States. Her website is purnamwellness.com. E-mail her for more information at dewestyoga@yahoo.com.

Melissa Williams

Melissa began her teacher training in 2003 at the Santa Barbara Yoga Center and finished just before she got married in 2004. She focuses on women's health issues, including eating disorders, pregnancy, and postpartum health. She is certified in pre- and postnatal yoga as well as children's yoga. Melissa lives in Louisville, Colorado, where she runs the Yoga Junction yoga studio. You can visit her at louisvilleyogajunction.com.

Margi Young

Margi is endlessly amazed at the joy and wonder of the human experience. Her curiosity began with a career in modern dance and only deepened the day she walked into OM Yoga Center where she felt like she had come home. She taught at OM for ten years and was a key player in the teacher training staff. She currently lives and teaches in the San Francisco Bay Area. Her website is margiyoung.com.

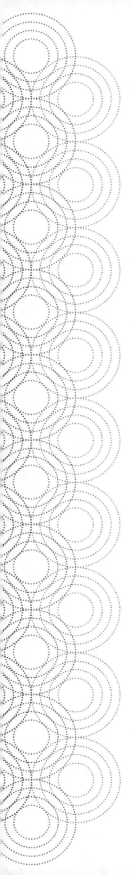

ABOUT THE AUTHOR

Linda Sparrowe has a long and varied career as a writer, editor, teacher, and mentor in the holistic healing arena, with a special emphasis on women's health and yoga. As the former editor-in-chief of *Yoga International* magazine, past managing editor of and long-time contributor to *Yoga Journal*, and featured expert in the films *YogaWoman* and *What Is Real? The Story of Jivamuki Yoga*, Linda has been instrumental in bringing the authentic voice of yoga to thousands of yoga teachers and practitioners who are ready to take their practice to the next level.

She has lent her writing and editing skills to a variety of book projects and has authored several books of her own, including *The Woman's Book of Yoga and Health: A Lifelong Guide to Wellness*; *Yoga for Healthy Bones*; and *Yoga for Healthy Menstruation* (all with Patricia Walden); *YOGA: A Yoga Journal Book*, a coffee-table book that chronicles the history of yoga and showcases more than 350 photographs (by David Martinez) of awe-inspiring yoga poses; and her latest one, *Yoga at Home: Inspiration for Creating Your Own Home Practice*.

She is on the advisory board of the Yoga and Body Image Coalition and contributed a chapter in the book *Yoga and Body Image* (Llewellyn Publications, 2014).

A long-time yoga teacher, Linda co-leads the Courageous Women, Fearless Living retreats for women touched by cancer—her heart's work. She mentors yoga teachers and often guest-teaches at teacher-training workshops. She has appeared on several radio shows, podcasts, and TV, gives talks on yoga in a variety of venues, and serves as an expert on yoga and women's health. She lives on the East Coast with her husband, Jim, and Redford, a very large, quite adorable golden retriever.

INDEX

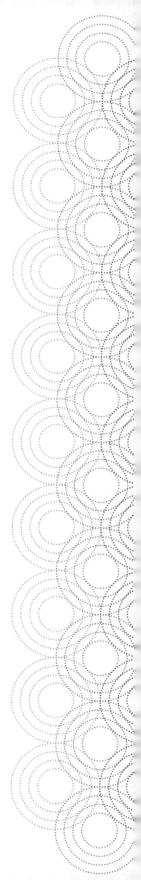

extended exhalation breathing, 214

Extended Puppy Pose (Uttana Shishosana), 22, 67

Extended Side-Angle Pose (Utthita Parsvakonasana), 33

Extended Triangle Pose (Utthita Trikonasana), 23, 35, 70, 130

"false labor," 147, 148

fatigue, 21

fatigue sequence, 22–26

fear and anxiety, managing, 115–19
   how to allay your fears, 116–17
   tips to calm a racing mind, 119

Figure Eights, 94

films, documentary, 223

Fire Log Pose (Agni Stambhasana), 55

first trimester, 1–4
   adjusting your yoga practice, 5
   challenges in, 12–15
   returning to the roots of practice, 7–12
   slowing down, 6–7
   staying strong, 5–6
   taking an internal inventory, 4
   See also specific topics

first trimester practice, 27–39

food, 57–58

food cravings, 58–59

forward bending
   after twenty weeks, 109
   seated, 38, 109–10

   See also Parivrtta Prasarita Padottanasana (Wide-Legged Standing Forward Bend) with Twist; Prasarita Padottanasana; Standing Forward Bend

forward extensions, standing, 108

fourth trimester challenges, 181–85
   getting your body back, 189–92
   how yoga can help, 185–87

fourth trimester practice, 187–89
   finding time for yoga, 208
   redefining your practice, 207–8

Franklin, Eric, 83, 85

friendships, 106

Garland Pose (Malasana), 37, 56, 74

Gaskin, Ina May
   methods, 151, 153,154
   philosophy 139, 141, 147, 149,

Gates, Janice, 9, 47, 61

Goddess Pose. *See* Parsva Utkata Konasana; Side-Stretching Goddess Pose; Utkata Konasana (Goddess Pose) Vinyasa

gratitude, 105–6

gravity-eliminating flow practice, 193–96

Half Downward-Facing Dog Pose (Ardha Adho Mukha Svanasana), 211

Half-Moon Pose (Ardha Chandrasana), 19, 34, 131